Patients, the Public and Priorities in Healthcare

Patients, the Public and Priorities in Healthcare

Edited by

PROFESSOR PETER LITTLEJOHNS
Clinical and Public Health Director
National Institute for Health and Clinical Excellence
Professor of Public Health
St George's University of London

and

PROFESSOR SIR MICHAEL RAWLINS
Chairman
National Institute for Health and Clinical Excellence

Foreword by

ALBERT WEALE
ESRC Professorial Fellow, Department of Government, University of Essex
Chair, Nuffield Council on Bioethics

Radcliffe Publishing
Oxford • New York

Radcliffe Publishing Ltd
18 Marcham Road
Abingdon
Oxon OX14 1AA
United Kingdom

www.radcliffe-oxford.com

Electronic catalogue and worldwide online ordering facility.

British Library Cataloguing in Publication Data

A catalogue record for this book is available from the British Library.

ISBN-13: 978 184619 387 3

The paper used for the text pages of this book is FSC certified. FSC (The Forest Stewardship Council) is an international network to promote responsible management of the world's forests.

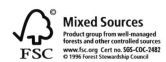

Mixed Sources
Product group from well-managed forests and other controlled sources
www.fsc.org Cert no. SGS-COC-2482
© 1996 Forest Stewardship Council

Copy-edited by Rachael Mayfield
Typeset by Pindar NZ, Auckland, New Zealand
Printed and bound by TJI Digital, Padstow, Cornwall, UK

Contents

Foreword

Sharing the costs of ill health is the mark of a civilised society. But even the most civilised society has to confront the limits of sharing. Some interventions are very expensive and their effect may vary across patients. Some people take more care of their own health than others. Treatments that look good in the laboratory turn out to be less effective in practice. Resources spent on the many can reduce care for the few. Prevention may be better than cure, but we need to balance money spent on prevention against the needs of those now suffering. In short, being prudent as well as civilised means that we have to think hard about the cost effectiveness of medical interventions.

In the UK, the body that does the hard thinking for us is NICE. Since 1999 it has aspired to give practicable and workable guidance through the mass of issues prompted by concerns for cost effective healthcare. In doing this it is has fostered various forms of public involvement, most obviously its Citizens Council, but also public consultations, workshops and transparency on its website.

But what is the point of public involvement? Reading these chapters makes it clear that some obvious answers will not stand up. Public involvement may not reduce controversy; recent decisions by NICE have been as controversial as any. Some say that public involvement allows otherwise suppressed voices to be heard, yet others allege that it gives more power to vocal groups well funded by industry. Public involvement may not lead to consensus because the experience of participants shows that some issues are so difficult and controversial that reasonable people will disagree as to how they are resolved. What is more, public involvement adds to the costs of decision making. What then exactly is the point?

Here is a possible reply. Public involvement of an open and transparent kind is the best way that we have found of channelling points of deep philosophical and political disagreement into civilised form. Evaluating cost effectiveness relies upon sound scientific and economic appraisal, but it also inevitably requires judgement about the values that a society should pursue. A democratic society makes any of its citizens qualified to judge on such issues, despite their complexity and controversy. Reading this volume will enable you, the reader, to assess how well NICE is acting as a means of fostering responsible public choice. I hope you profit from its chapters as much as I have.

Albert Weale
ESRC Professorial Fellow, Department of Government,
University of Essex
Chair, Nuffield Council on Bioethics
October 2009

Preface

In most countries there is a move to encourage patients and the public to become active partners in a new relationship with healthcare professionals. The aim is to enable an informed public to make 'health choices' to reduce their risk of disease, to manage chronic conditions and to make appropriate end-of-life decisions. Increasingly patients are also getting involved in making decisions about the prioritisation of healthcare, alongside policy makers and politicians.

The National Institute for Health and Clinical Excellence (NICE) has sought to integrate patients and the public in all of its decisions. NICE's remit has expanded over the 10 years that it has existed and as a result, it has experience of involving patients in most aspects of healthcare.

All NICE decision-making bodies have patient representatives and all national patient groups can submit evidence and respond to draft guidance though a process of consultation. NICE has a patient and public involvement programme to support patients in making this contribution to its guidance and this provides training, support and evaluation. In order to understand the social values that are needed to underpin its advisory body decisions, NICE established a Citizens Council that consists of 30 people drawn from the general public.

During the years that NICE has built up these programmes it has been approached by a range of national and international organisations and governments to describe and share its experiences in establishing and running the Citizens Council, and encouraging and supporting patient involvement. This book is part of NICE's response to these expressions of interest and it has three aims.

The first is to provide an up-to-date 'position statement' on the Citizens Council, explaining why it was established; how it has been run; its impact; the lessons learnt and proposed future developments. It sets the Council in the context of a national health policy organisation and how it determines the values underpinning its decision making.

The second aim of the book is to describe the various opportunities for patients to interact with NICE and how their views are carefully taken into account.

The final aim is to provide an opportunity for a national and international perspective on some of the novel issues facing the interaction between patients, the public and the provision of healthcare. For this we thank Sir Iain Chalmers and his colleagues, and Marthe Gold and Norman Daniels.

Professor Peter Littlejohns
Clinical and Public Health Director
National Institute for Health and Clinical Excellence
Professor of Public Health, St George's University of London

Professor Sir Michael Rawlins
Chairman
National Institute for Health and Clinical Excellence
October 2009

Contributors

Lizzie Amis
Project Manager, Patient and Public Involvement Programme
National Institute for Health and Clinical Excellence

Elizabeth Barnett
ex-Research Fellow
Faculty of Health and Social Care, The Open University
Now retraining in psychotherapy

Anne Brice
Associate Director, National Knowledge Service

Brian Brown
Citizens Council Member 2002–6

Iain Chalmers
Coordinator, UK Database of Uncertainties about the Effects of Treatments

Emma Chambers
Project Manager, Patient and Public Involvement Programme
National Institute for Health and Clinical Excellence

Jane Cowl
Programme Manager, Patient and Public Involvement Programme
National Institute for Health and Clinical Excellence

Professor Norman Daniels
Professor of Ethics and Population Health
Harvard School of Public Health

Professor Celia Davies
Emeritus Professor of Health Care
The Open University

Mark Fenton
Editor, UK Database of Uncertainties about the Effects of Treatments

Dr Marcia Kelson
Associate Director, Patient and Public Involvement Programme
National Institute for Health and Clinical Excellence

Professor Marthe Gold
Professor of Community Health and Social Medicine
City College of New York

Professor Peter Littlejohns
Clinical and Public Health Director
National Institute for Health and Clinical Excellence
Professor of Public Health
St George's University of London

Laura Norburn
Project Manager, Patient and Public Involvement Programme
National Institute for Health and Clinical Excellence

Ela Pathak-Sen
Director, Commotion UK

Professor Sir Michael Rawlins
Chairman
National Institute for Health and Clinical Excellence

Victoria Thomas
Programme Manager, Patient and Public Involvement Programme
National Institute for Health and Clinical Excellence

Margaret Wetherell
Professor of Social Psychology, Open University
Director, Economic and Social Research Council Programme on Identities and
Social Action

Figures and tables

FIGURES

TABLES

Glossary

Advisory bodies NICE's advisory bodies develop NICE guidance. The advisory bodies (September 2009) are: the three technology appraisal committees, the Interventional Procedures Advisory Committee, the subject-specific guideline development groups and their guideline review panels, the Public Health Interventions Advisory Committee and the subject-specific public health programme development groups.

Beneficence The obligation to benefit individuals.

Bioethics The ethics of medical and biological research and practice.

Carer Someone, who, without payment, provides help and support to a partner, child, relative, friend or neighbour, who could not manage without their help, because of age, physical or mental illness, addiction or disability.

Citizen capture When the opinions of a member of the public are unduly influenced by another individual or group without the member of the public being aware of it.

Citizens Council The Citizens Council brings the views of the public to NICE decision making about guidance on the promotion of good health and the prevention and treatment of ill health. Comprising 30 people drawn from all walks of life, the Citizens Council tackles challenging questions about values – such as fairness and need.

Clinical effectiveness The extent to which a specific treatment or intervention, when used under usual or everyday conditions, has a beneficial effect on the course or outcome of disease compared to no treatment or other routine care.

Clinical efficacy The extent to which a specific treatment or intervention, under ideally controlled conditions, has a beneficial effect on the course or outcome of disease compared with no treatment or other routine care.

Clinical guideline NICE guidance on the treatment and care, in the NHS, of people with a specific disease or condition.

Clinician A healthcare professional providing patient care; for example, a doctor, nurse or physiotherapist.

Consultees Organisations invited to take part in a technology appraisal. Consultee organisations include: national groups representing patients and carers; bodies representing healthcare professionals; manufacturers of the health technology being appraised.

Cost effectiveness Value for money; a specific healthcare treatment is said to be 'cost effective' if it gives a greater health gain than could be achieved by using the resources in other ways.

Cost-effectiveness analysis A type of economic evaluation comparing the costs and the effects on health of different treatments. Health effects are measured in 'health-related units', for example, the cost of preventing one additional heart attack.

Cost-utility analysis A form of cost-effectiveness analysis where a treatment is assessed in terms of its ability to both extend life and to improve the quality of life. The unit of measurement is called a quality-adjusted life year (QALY).

Dialogue across difference A discussion, debate and sharing of different views. The emphasis is for people with conflicting viewpoints to attempt to understand and come to terms with each other's views, rather than 'win' the debate.

Directions Legally binding instructions to NICE (or other NHS bodies), from the Secretary of State, on the conduct of its affairs.

Distributive justice The fair and consistent allocation of goods or services (including healthcare) to society.

Effectiveness *See* 'Clinical effectiveness'.

Efficacy *See* 'Clinical efficacy'.

Efficiency In healthcare, efficiency involves using the available resources in a manner that maximises the health of the population as a whole.

Establishment orders (NICE's) The legal instruments establishing NICE, authorising its legal powers, and indicating the arrangements for its governance.

Ethnographic study An observational study of a particular culture, society or community.

Evidence Information on which a decision or guidance is based. Evidence is obtained from a range of sources including randomised controlled trials, observational studies and expert opinion (of clinical professionals and/or patients).

Experiential learning Learning derived from experience.

Generalisability The extent to which the results of a study conducted in a particular patient population and/or a specific context will apply for another population and/or in a different context.

Guideline development group A group of healthcare professionals, patients, carers and technical staff who develop the recommendations for a NICE clinical guideline.

Health-related quality of life A combination of an individual's physical, mental and social well-being; not merely the absence of disease.

Health technologies New and existing drugs, devices, treatments, surgical procedures and therapies designed to prevent and treat disease and/or improve rehabilitation and long-term care.

Incremental cost-effectiveness ratio (ICER) The ratio of the difference in the mean costs of a technology compared with the next best alternative to the difference in the mean outcomes.

Interventional procedure An interventional procedure is a procedure used for diagnosis or treatment that involves making a cut or hole in the patient's body, entry into a body cavity or using electromagnetic radiation (including X-rays or lasers).

Interventional Procedures Advisory Committee The independent committee that advises NICE on whether an interventional procedure is safe enough and works well enough to be used in the NHS.

NICE guidance NICE produces guidance in three main areas: health technologies, focusing on the use of new and existing drugs, devices, therapies and surgical procedures; clinical practice, relating to appropriate treatment for specific diseases and conditions; and public health, involving the promotion of good health and prevention of ill health.

Non-maleficence An obligation not to inflict either physical or psychological harm.

Open space technology A method to run meetings of groups of any size. It is a self-organising process; participants construct the agenda and schedule during the meeting itself.

Orphan drugs Drugs indicated for rare conditions or diseases (those that occur in fewer than 1 in 2000 of the population).

Outcome measure A measure of the degree of success obtained from the treatment or care of a disease or condition.

Partners Council The Council consists of individuals nominated by groups representing patient and public interests, health professional bodies, academic institutions, NHS management, healthcare-quality organisations, industry and trade unions. It provides a forum for the exchange of ideas, concepts and future plans and provides NICE with the views of a range of organisations that have an interest in its work.

Patient and Public Involvement Programme (PPIP) A dedicated team within NICE that develops and supports opportunities for patient, carer and public involvement.

Primary research Original research conducted to collect new data to answer a research question.

Public health The science and art of preventing disease, prolonging life and promoting health through organised efforts of society.

Public Health Interventions Advisory Committee An independent advisory body that produces recommendations for NICE on the use of discrete activities (interventions) that help to reduce people's risk of developing a disease or condition or help to promote or maintain a healthy lifestyle. Examples of interventions include giving advice, providing services or providing support on specific topics: for example, giving advice in GP practices to encourage exercise, providing a needle exchange scheme for injecting drug users, providing support on breastfeeding for new mothers.

Public Health Programme Development Group An independent advisory body that produces recommendations for NICE on broad actions for the promotion of good health and the prevention of ill health. This guidance may focus on a topic, such as smoking, or on a particular population, such as young people, or on a particular setting, such as the workplace.

Quality-adjusted life year (QALY) A measure of health outcome that looks at both length of life and quality of life. QALYs are calculated by estimating the years of life remaining for a patient following a particular care pathway and weighting each year with a quality-of-life score (on a zero to one scale). One QALY is equal to one year of life in perfect health, or two years at 50% health, and so on.

Qualitative research A method of research that explores and tries to understand people's beliefs, experiences, attitudes, behaviour and interactions. It generates non-numerical data. It is more subjective than quantitative research (*see* 'Quantitative research') and is often exploratory and open ended. Examples include in-depth interviews, focus groups, documentary analysis and participant observation.

Quality of life *See* 'Health-related quality of life'.

Quantitative research A method of research that uses statistical methods to count and measure outcomes from a study. The outcomes are usually objective and predetermined. A large number of participants are usually required to ensure that the results are statistically significant.

Stakeholder An organisation with an interest in a topic on which NICE is developing a clinical guideline or piece of public health guidance. Stakeholders may be: manufacturers of drugs or equipment; national patient and carer organisations; NHS organisations; organisations representing healthcare professionals.

Secondary research This involves the summary, collation and/or synthesis of existing research.

Systematic review Research that identifies and analyses the full range of good quality scientific studies that have been carried out to answer the same question.

Technology *See* 'Health technology'.

Technology appraisal committee An independent advisory body that reviews evidence to produce recommendations for NICE on the use of technologies (new and existing drugs, devices, treatments, surgical procedures and therapies) in the NHS.

Technology appraisal guidance NICE recommendations on the use of new and existing drugs, devices, treatments, surgical procedures and therapies within the NHS in England and Wales.

Ultra-orphan drug A term used by NICE to describe a drug used for very rare conditions or diseases that occur in fewer than 1 in 50 000 of the population; it also covers pharmaceutical interventions for which there are no other known or possible uses.

Utility A measure of the strength of a person's preference for a specific health state in relation to alternative health states. The utility scale assigns numerical values on a scale from 0 (death) to 1 (optimal or 'perfect' health). Health states can be considered worse than death and thus have a negative value.

CHAPTER 1

The establishment of NICE

Peter Littlejohns

NICE is an independent organisation responsible for providing national guidance on promoting good health and preventing and treating ill health in England and Wales. It was established as a special health authority in 1999 to offer National Health Service (NHS) professionals advice on how to provide their patients with the highest attainable standards of care and to reduce variation in the quality of care. Specifically, NICE aims to speed the uptake of interventions that are both clinically and cost effective (i.e. that work and are value for money). It also aims to encourage more equitable access to healthcare, provide better and more rational use of available resources by focusing on the most cost-effective interventions, and encourage the creation and dissemination of new and innovative technologies.

Since its inception NICE has been controversial.[1,2] This was inevitable because for the first time a national organisation was explicitly stating that the healthcare system could not afford all the interventions that could benefit individual patients. Treatments needed to be prioritised according to the extra value that they provided to patients compared with existing practice. The approach that NICE took was based on a number of key principles.

➤ All of its guidance should be based on the best available evidence.
➤ The process should be as open and transparent as possible.
➤ The process should be inclusive: any stakeholder likely to be affected by its guidance should be part of the development of that guidance, either by being a member of one of the independent advisory bodies or through participating in open consultations.

All NICE advisory bodies contain healthcare academics, professionals, industry representatives, patients and where appropriate, the general public. Most of NICE's advisory bodies now meet in public. Over the years NICE has developed particular expertise in patient and public involvement. It has established a designated patient and public involvement programme and a Citizens Council, which consists of members of the public who consider the nature of social values underpinning NICE guidance.

Over the 10 years it has existed, NICE has been invited to take on a range of new responsibilities. A major development occurred in 2005 when its remit was expanded to include health promotion and disease prevention.[3] This followed an independent review of policies to achieve cost-effective improvements in the health of the English population and reductions in health inequalities. The review was commissioned by the UK's treasury department and resulted in a white paper on public health policy.[4,5]

NICE currently has four programmes that produce guidance (*see* Table 1.1). These are: technology appraisals, clinical guidelines, interventional procedures and public health guidance. Most programmes take both effectiveness (how well an intervention works) and cost effectiveness (how well it works in relation to how much it costs) into account.

TABLE 1.1: NICE guidance programmes.

NICE programme	Provides guidance on	What the guidance takes into account
Technology appraisals	The use of health technologies, which include: ● pharmaceuticals ● medical devices ● diagnostics ● surgical and other procedures ● health promotion tools	Clinical effectiveness and cost effectiveness
Clinical guidelines	The appropriate treatment and care of patients with specific diseases and conditions	Clinical effectiveness and cost effectiveness
Interventional procedures	The safety of an interventional procedure and how well it works	Clinical efficacy and safety of the intervention It does not take cost effectiveness into account
Public health guidance	Activities to promote a healthy lifestyle and prevent ill health (for example, giving advice to encourage exercise, or providing support to encourage mothers to breastfeed)	Effectiveness and cost effectiveness of public health activities

Currently, NICE has 311 full-time staff with an annual budget of £35 million. It has offices based in London and, since 2005, also in Manchester. However, its guidance development is supported through a series of directly commissioned

National Collaborating Centres and university-based academic units funded through the National Institute for Health Research (NIHR), the body responsible for funding NHS research in England. This means that more than 2000 individuals (excluding external stakeholders) are involved in developing guidance at any one time. Following a national review during 2007/08 to establish a 10-year vision of the NHS by Lord Darzi, the functions of NICE will expand further.[6]

NICE has now produced guidance in most fields of healthcare and public health. Although NICE does not have responsibility for ensuring that its guidance is put into practice it soon became apparent that more support for implementation in the NHS was required. In 2004 an implementation directorate was established to support guidance implementation through a series of education and liaison functions. Support tools (including costing templates) are now issued with each guidance document.

CONTROVERSIAL DECISIONS

While much of NICE guidance has been welcomed, it is inevitable that both the general and professional media concentrate on the controversial nature of those recommendations that limit access to cost-ineffective treatment. NICE guidance recommendations are rarely completely negative. However, they may recommend treatment for a more-targeted group of patients than is represented in the full licensed indications of a drug. For example in the field of oncology where decisions have generated the most consistent controversy, between 1999 and 2009 NICE made 76 decisions in 47 appraisals for cancer agents. A decision to not recommend for any licensed indication was made in only 13% of appraisals (10 decisions). In 46% of appraisals (35 decisions) the guidance recommended use in line with their licensed indications, and for 28% of appraisals (21 decisions) the recommendations were restricted to certain patient groups (usually on the basis of cost effectiveness). In 8% of appraisals (six decisions) recommendations were made for the drug to be used in a research setting only, and in 5% of appraisals (four decisions), industry declined to submit evidence.

Perhaps due in part to NICE's continuing argument that cost effectiveness is determined by two factors, that is, if you cannot improve effectiveness then cost needs to be reduced, manufacturers have started to explore ways in which their drug can be made available in a cost-effective way to the NHS. These 'access schemes' have required negotiations with and approval of the Department of Health before being referred to NICE for consideration. The first cancer guidance incorporating this approach concerned bortezomib for multiple myeloma. A similar approach was taken with ranibizumab for the treatment of macular degeneration where industry pays for treatment after the initial 14 injections.

Since its inception NICE has maintained that efficiency in terms of cost effectiveness, and accounting for opportunity costs were key determinants of assessing value. However, other factors such as fairness and reducing health inequalities are also important. These other 'values' are encapsulated in the document *Social Value Judgements: principles for the development of NICE guidance*, first published in 2005 and further refined in the second edition published in 2008.[7] This document forms the basis of NICE's advice to its advisory bodies on how to apply social value judgements when making decisions. The eight social value principles were formulated through a series of workshops involving ethicists and moral philosophers as well as reports from the Citizens Council.

NICE uses the quality-adjusted life year (QALY) as the main health outcome measure. This unit combines both quantity (length) of life and health-related quality of life into a single measure of health gain. A review of guidance decisions during the first few years has indicated that NICE's threshold for cost effectiveness lies in the range of £20 000 to £30 000 per QALY. However, NICE's independent advisory bodies have always had latitude to recommend technologies for which the cost effectiveness is above the upper range, providing there is a strong case to do so.

In 2006 the Office of Fair Trading (the UK body responsible for ensuring that markets work for consumers) produced a report that suggested the existing scheme for pricing drugs in the UK was not beneficial to the NHS. It advocated a 'value-based' approach to pricing on the basis of assessments similar to those undertaken by NICE.[8] In 2008 the Department of Health terminated the existing Pharmaceutical Price Regulation Scheme (PPRS) and negotiated a new process with the industry, which was agreed and published in December 2008.[9] In the new PPRS agreement, NICE has a role in providing information on the cost effectiveness of new drugs. The single technology appraisal programme, introduced as a means of ensuring that NICE appraisals can be published as close to the licensing of new drugs as possible, will need to expand as a consequence.

Another major development relevant to NICE's appraisal programme was the report by the Department of Health's National Clinical Director for Cancer, Professor Mike Richards, in 2008.[10] Following public concern, he was invited to undertake a review of the status of ongoing NHS treatments if patients decided to buy drugs that were not recommended by NICE or funded by their primary care trust (PCT) – so-called 'top-up' payments. The Department of Health accepted the recommendations of this report in their entirety. This meant that if patients wished to pay for treatments not approved by NICE or funded by their PCT they would no longer have to also pay for the rest of their NHS treatment. The acceptance of this principle was in part based on NICE being able to issue guidance on drugs close to their licensing.

Alongside the report by Professor Richards, NICE has been exploring methods to capture patients' values on treatments that extend life in situations of very limited life expectance. These explorations have focused on drugs that are not cures but, nonetheless, extend life. In conjunction with the NIHR, NICE has previously commissioned a series of research projects to assess whether society would assign the same value to quality of life and life expectancy (measured as QALYs) under all circumstances. Citizens Council reports, as well as the commissioned research, suggest that this assumption may not fit in with society's view and that society may well place greater importance on some circumstances, such as severe disease, or disease in children. While the methodological research suggests that 'weighting' should be considered, it does not provide a definitive list of what these circumstances should be or by how much. In January 2009 NICE issued further advice to the technology appraisal advisory bodies around their explorations of cost effectiveness of end-of-life interventions with consideration to this important issue.

As a public body NICE is subject to judicial review and despite the controversial nature of its guidance, it didn't receive a legal challenge for the first eight years of its existence. In the last two years there have been three legal challenges. The results have, in general, supported NICE processes, although some changes have had to be made to the appraisal process to allow stakeholders to scrutinise the cost-effectiveness model. No guidance has been materially affected by the court's decisions.

HOW NICE MANAGES UNCERTAINTY

The UK has traditionally been internationally excellent in undertaking basic research but less skilled at translating that work into routine practice. To address this issue, Sir David Cooksey undertook a major review of UK health research in 2006. Sir Cooksey called for more collaboration between key stakeholders, including the Medical Research Council (MRC), NHS Research and Development, NICE and industry.[11] Sir Cooksey proposed a series of actions to ensure that publicly-funded health research was carried out in the most effective and efficient way, resulting in a timely translation of research findings into health and economic benefits.

The most important recommendations from NICE's perspective were recommendations for enhancing drug development and the uptake of clinically effective and cost-effective new technologies. The proposed mechanism for this was to adopt a more proactive approach in the NHS and create a new partnership between government, regulators and industry to pilot a new drug development 'pathway'. In response NICE has developed two main work streams. The first, working with industry through a new 'scientific advice programme' to ensure that the appropriate data is collected at an early stage in drug development, and the second, a series of proposals to support the collection of data at a national level and ensure that the evidence gaps identified by NICE are filled.[12,13] NICE is working with the NIHR and MRC to facilitate this development. NICE has also led the exploration of a 'fit-for-purpose' approach to the collection of data rather than the traditional hierarchical approach.[14]

NICE AND THE NHS 10-YEAR VISION

The report on the future of the NHS, published in 2008 to coincide with the 60th anniversary of the NHS, restated a clear commitment to a publicly funded healthcare system and makes quality of care its driving force.[6] It describes a vision of the NHS that is: fair – equally available to all; personalised – tailored to the wants of each individual; effective – focused on delivering outcomes for patients; and safe. It emphasises the need to make the best use of resources to provide the most effective care, and reinforces the messages set out in the operating framework for England 2008/09 by focusing on the needs and preferences of patients, improving patient care and emphasising the importance of commissioning.

The report recognises the role of NICE in setting standards and in providing guidance on clinical and cost effectiveness. As a result, all NICE's existing programmes were expanded to take on additional work, such as a programme evaluating diagnostic tests. New programmes were also created as a result, such as NHS Evidence (a new portal for NHS staff to access information) and the evidence base underpinning the Quality and Outcomes Framework (QOF), the system of financial incentives to improve primary care services within the contract between general practitioners and the NHS.

The role of the main health regulator has always been important to NICE in supporting the implementation of its guidance. April 2009 saw the birth of the third organisation that NICE has worked with in the last 10 years. The first was the Commission for Health Improvement and, over the past three years, NICE has worked with the Healthcare Commission to inform its annual review of the performance of NHS organisations against national standards established in 2004.[15] In April 2009 a new body, the Care Quality Commission, took on the responsibility for regulating both health and adult social care.

The principles for the future model of regulation were published in October 2007. They propose a set of registration requirements that focus on safety and quality and cover all health and social care provider organisations, whether NHS, private or third sector. The requirements, which the Care Quality Commission will consult on during 2009, will be based in part on the 'core' standards within the current national standards, that is, those representing the minimum acceptable performance. The Care Quality Commission will be responsible for registering providers that comply with these requirements. Further changes to the system of standards, particularly those to be used for encouraging improvements in performance within the NHS performance management system, are expected in 2009. These represent a potentially significant change in the way that NICE guidance is positioned in the NHS. NICE will be working with the Care Quality Commission and the Department of Health to clarify the relationship between the new registration standards and the quality standards that NICE has been asked to produce.

THE NEXT 10 YEARS

NICE is now firmly established as part of the NHS landscape. Like the NHS itself it is praised and criticised in equal measure. Whether everybody would go as far as the editor of the *BMJ* and call NICE a 'national treasure' is debatable in itself.[16] However, as the *BMJ* editorial concludes, 'NICE needs critical friends'. Despite dissension over individual decisions NICE has managed to create a broad consensus that prioritisation of healthcare is necessary and that an open and evidenced approach is probably the best. NICE's strategy for achieving this has been based on involving thousands of patients, professionals, academics and industry representatives in developing guidance over the years.

A lot has been learnt in the first 10 years and there is still more to learn. NICE was created and has functioned at a time of unprecedented growth in NHS funds. In the last 10 years the NHS budget has grown by an annual 6.1%. This year it will rise by 5.5%. From April 2011, spending will rise by only 1%. However, this was before the current financial storm occurred so times ahead may be even leaner. NICE already advises the NHS on how to 'disinvest' from cost-ineffective practice, but it is likely that this work will need more prominence in the future.[17,18]

NICE methods have been carefully scrutinised by many other countries and in response, NICE has established an international consultancy capacity to share its experience of seeking to ensure a fair allocation of healthcare resources for all.[19] The consultancy works mainly with countries that are just establishing the capacity to evaluate the value of healthcare interventions, but, in addition, NICE has regular meetings with similar organisations in countries that have already established this capacity, such as France and Germany. These meetings allow a sharing of methodological challenges and ways to respond to them. Of course everyone is watching the US with keen interest to see how Obama's new drive to create the capacity to assess 'comparative effectiveness' will affect the biggest health market in the world.

REFERENCES

1 Littlejohns P, Barnett D, Longson C. The cancer technology appraisal programme of the UK's National Institute for Clinical Excellence. *Lancet Oncol.* 2003; 4(4): 242–50.
2 Littlejohns P, Garner S, Doyle N, *et al.* 10 years of NICE: still growing and still controversial. *Lancet Oncol.* 2009; **10**(4): 417–24.

3 Littlejohns P, Kelly M. The changing face of NICE: the same but different. *Lancet.* 2005; **366**(9488): 791–4.

4 Wanless D. *Securing Good Health for the Whole Population: final report.* London: HMSO; February 2004.

5 Department of Health. *Choosing Health: making healthy choices easier.* Cm. 6374. London: Department of Health; 2004.

6 Darzi A. *High Quality Care for All: NHS next stage review final report.* Cm. 7432. London: Department of Health; 2008.

7 National Institute for Health and Clinical Excellence. *Social Value Judgements: principles for the development of NICE guidance.* 2nd ed. London: NIHCE; 2008. Available at: www.nice.org.uk/media/C18/30/SVJ2PUBLICATION2008.pdf (accessed 22 September 2009).

8 Office of Fair Trading. *Pharmaceutical Price Regulation Scheme: an OFT market study.* London: Office of Fair Trading; 2007.

9 Department of Health. *Pharmaceutical Price Regulation Scheme.* London: Department of Health; 2008.

10 Richards M. *Improving Access to Medicines for NHS Patients: a report for the Secretary of State for Health.* London: Department of Health; 2008.

11 Cooksey D. *A Review of UK Health Research Funding.* London: The Stationery Office; 2006.

12 Chalkidou K, Lord J, Fischer A, *et al.* Evidence-based decision making: when should we wait for more information? *Health Aff (Millwood).* 2008; **27**(6): 1642–53.

13 Chalkidou K, Walley T, Culyer A, *et al.* Evidence-informed evidence-making. *J Health Serv Res Policy.* 2008; **13**(3): 167–73.

14 Rawlins MD. De testimonio: on the evidence for decisions about the use of therapeutic interventions. *Lancet.* 2008; **372**(9656): 2152–61.

15 Department of Health. *Standards for Better Health.* London: Department of Health; 2004.

16 Godlee F. NICE at 10. *BMJ.* 2009; **338**: b344.

17 Pearson S, Littlejohns P. Reallocating resources: how should the National Institute for Health and Clinical Excellence guide disinvestment efforts in the NHS? *J Health Serv Res Policy.* 2007; **12**(3): 160–5.

18 National Institute for Health and Clinical Excellence. *Optimal Practice Review: recommendation reminders.* London: NIHCE; 2009. Available at: www.nice.org.uk/usingguidance/optimalpracticereviewrecommendationreminders/optimal_practice_review_recommendation_reminders.jsp (accessed 22 September 2009).

19 Hawkes N. NICE goes global. *BMJ.* 2009; **338**: b103.

CHAPTER 2

NICE's commitment to patient, carer and public involvement

Marcia Kelson

The views of patients or service users, their carers, and the public matter to NICE. We seek to involve them, as well as doctors, nurses, other healthcare professionals and managers in every aspect of our work. In doing so, NICE aims to produce guidance that addresses patient/carer/public issues, reflects their views and meets their healthcare needs.

Patients, carers and the public can get involved in NICE's work by commenting on draft versions of our guidance. There are also opportunities to get involved more directly in the work NICE does to produce its guidance. This includes contributing to making the decisions (sometimes difficult ones) that have to be taken when recommending that the NHS should offer or refuse specific treatments.

PRINCIPLES OF PATIENT, CARER AND PUBLIC INVOLVEMENT

The principles that NICE follows with regard to involving the public in its work are to
➤ produce clinical guidance for the NHS that is patient centred
➤ produce public health guidance that focuses on the public's needs
➤ provide opportunities for patients, carers and the public to contribute alongside health professionals and industry (companies producing drugs, medical devices and diagnostic equipment) to the collection of evidence that informs our guidance
➤ involve patients, carers and the public in NICE decision making
➤ support patients, carers and the public who contribute to the production of NICE guidance

➤ produce versions of NICE guidance written specifically for patients, carers and the public

➤ work with patients, carers, patient organisations and the media to publicise our recommendations to help people access the treatment they are entitled to

➤ review the processes and methods used to involve patients, carers and the public in NICE's work.

NICE'S PATIENT AND PUBLIC INVOLVEMENT PROGRAMME

NICE has, from its inception, made a firm commitment to involve patients, carers and the public in its activities. This commitment is formally set out in its patient and public involvement policy and through the resourcing of a dedicated team, the Patient and Public Involvement Programme (PPIP). The PPIP develops and supports opportunities for patients, carers and members of the public (organisations and individuals) to contribute to the range of activities carried out by NICE.

The PPIP currently employs nine members of staff who:

➤ advise NICE and its partners on alternative methods for securing involvement

➤ work with other NICE staff to develop and integrate involvement opportunities in all NICE activities

➤ identify patient, carer, community and other lay organisations that may be interested in contributing to NICE work programmes, so that they can be invited to participate

➤ facilitate the recruitment of individual patients, carers, community members and members of the public to NICE advisory bodies

➤ develop and provide ongoing training and support to lay members of NICE advisory bodies

➤ work with patient, carer and voluntary organisations to encourage and facilitate their engagement in NICE processes

➤ work with equality groups to identify opportunities for their involvement, increase diversity in the types of national organisations that engage with NICE and promote diversity in the lay membership of NICE advisory bodies

➤ promote the dissemination and uptake of NICE guidance for local patients and communities by working with organisations and groups that have a statutory responsibility for patient and public involvement in the wider NHS, such as primary care trusts, patient advice and liaison services and local involvement networks

➤ carry out or commission projects to evaluate the effectiveness of the opportunities that exist at NICE for patient, carer and public involvement

➤ work with local, national and international organisations to promote patient, carer and public involvement in activities influenced by the availability of NICE guidance.

OPPORTUNITIES FOR INVOLVEMENT

Opportunities for lay involvement exist at all key stages of NICE activity and take several forms.

➤ **Lay membership of NICE advisory bodies.** All NICE advisory bodies are expected to include at least two lay members (often more) who are recruited through open advertising. Successful applicants are those who most closely meet the criteria set out in the job description and person specification produced by the PPIP and the relevant NICE team(s) for each advisory body.

➤ **Consultation with national organisations that represent the interests of patients, carers, communities and the public.** Organisations interested in NICE consultations include specific groups for health conditions, organisations representing the interests of specific client groups (for example, groups representing children, older people, people with disabilities, people from different ethnic groups) and groups that focus on public health issues (for example transport or lifestyle choices). Organisations are regularly consulted in the development and review of NICE processes, and at key stages of guidance development. Many national patient- and voluntary organisations also provide valuable support by publicising and disseminating NICE guidance to a wider patient and public constituency and by promoting the uptake and implementation of NICE guidance at national and local levels.

➤ **Workshops or surveys.** These canvass the views of patients or the public to inform specific initiatives.

➤ **Deliberative consultation with the NICE Citizens Council.** This is a NICE initiative where 30 members of the public meet together twice a year to provide a public view on social and ethical issues that impact on how NICE carries out its work.

➤ **Information provision.** All NICE guidance has versions written for a patient/public audience to describe what NICE has recommended.

➤ **Patients involved in NICE (PIN) Group.**

COMMENTARY ON OPPORTUNITIES FOR PATIENT AND PUBLIC INVOLVEMENT AT NICE
Views from the outside

There is a growing body of literature on the role and impact of NICE's Citizens Council whose members' deliberations inform NICE's social value judgements.

However, literature focusing specifically on opportunities for patient and public involvement in the actual development of NICE guidance is more limited, and research evaluating these opportunities and their impact even more so.

NICE itself has published articles describing the opportunities for patient and public involvement and commissioned a study to be carried out by an independent researcher to evaluate patient and carer membership of its first 20 clinical guidelines.[1-4]

The chair of a guideline development group, Professor Richard Baker, has described the impact of patient involvement on the development of a clinical guideline on referral for suspected cancer.[5] Professor Baker noted the involvement of patients through guideline development groups and the formal consultation processes that take place during guideline development. He also referred to the inclusion of recommendations specifically concerned with patients' preferences and needs, and the provision of guidelines in a format specifically for patients. Professor Baker believes NICE guidelines are 'contributing to the creation of an NHS culture which values patient involvement'.

External commentaries include reviews of NICE's work by the World Health Organization, which commented favourably on opportunities for stakeholder involvement, including patients and the public.[6,7]

Other publications have focused on opportunities for involving patients, carers and the public in the development of NICE health technology appraisals guidance. Pauline Quennell examined the interaction of patient organisations with NICE during the first years of its existence.[8,9] To form her conclusions she used unstructured interviews with patient/carer representatives from NICE committees and those with an interest in NICE technology appraisals, her observation of NICE's Board and Partners Council, and the analysis of documentary evidence. Quennell found that most interviewees felt that the patient voice had been strengthened in NICE's structures and appraisal process. However, Quennell did voice concerns about the relative weightings of patient and scientific evidence, and perceptions by patient groups that their submissions of evidence had only a marginal impact.

Mark Duckenfield and Dwijen Rangekar explored the extent to which patient groups presented patient experts to attend as witnesses at appraisal committee meetings during the period of 1999–2003.[10] Duckenfield found that the numbers of patient and clinical experts were comparable. While acknowledging that measuring access is not the same as measuring influence, he concluded that patient groups were representing the medical interests of their members in a sophisticated fashion. Sir Iain Chalmers, however, has argued that patient organisations need to be more transparent about their relationships with and funding by the pharmaceutical industry.[11]

A report by the Mentor UK Youth Involvement Project documented the impact of public involvement on two pieces of NICE guidance.[12] These were *Interventions in Schools to Prevent and Reduce Alcohol Use Among Children and Young People* (NICE public health guidance 7)[13] and *Community-Based Interventions to Reduce Substance Misuse Among Vulnerable and Disadvantaged Children and Young People* (NICE public health guidance 4).[14] The authors identified how young people aged 12–20 influenced the guidance with the feedback they provided on the draft recommendations. Examples include changes to the wording of recommendations and the definition of the group of young people to be targeted, and the inclusion of additional recommendations to reflect a wider range of influences on young people's behaviour.

Not everyone is convinced that patient involvement is a good thing for NICE. Professor Robin Ferner and Sarah McDowell argued that NICE appraisals should be insulated from external pressure.[15] While noting that it is understandable that patients whose illnesses provide strong motivation to obtain a share of NHS resources wish their voices to be heard, Professor Ferner and McDowell cite further studies that criticise patient group input because they share a common interest with drug companies in promoting access to specific treatments that others will pay for.[16] They also cite concerns that patients may act as conduits for drug companies to promote their products and lobby for increased access to new drugs.[17,18]

Views from patient organisations

The most complete single collection of information on patient organisations' views of NICE can be found in the written submissions made to the Health Select Committee inquiry into NICE in 2007.[19] The focus of this, the second inquiry into NICE, was to consider:
➤ why NICE's decisions are increasingly being challenged
➤ whether public confidence in NICE is waning, and if so why
➤ NICE's evaluation process, and whether any particular groups are disadvantaged by the process.

There were 92 written submissions, of which 35% were submitted by patient organisations covering a range of constituencies including long-term conditions, cancer and maternity/gynaecology.

Five further submissions were submitted by individuals who identified themselves as patients or patient advocates but with no specific organisational affiliation.

There was overall, but by no means universal, acceptance that there is a role for NICE and approval of some, but not all of its methods, including methods for patient input. Here are two examples of comments:

'NICE plays a critical role in ensuring that NHS treatment is equitable, cost effective and of a uniformly high standard.'

'[NICE] guidance is often negative and flies in the face of the medical evidence supporting the efficacy of the treatments they are appraising . . . their decisions seem to be based solely on grounds of cost not efficacy.'

The majority of comments related to the development and implementation of NICE's guidance, predominantly but not exclusively its technology appraisal guidance. Issues raised included:

➤ the extent to which the research evidence and other evidence considered by NICE addresses issues that are important to patients, for example patient experiences/preferences and outcomes, such as quality of life

➤ concern that quality of life measures have often been determined by professionals and do not reflect the issues that patients consider most important

➤ concerns about the impact of patient submissions to NICE and the weighting that NICE advisory bodies place on patient evidence

➤ the opportunities for stakeholder (including patient) input

➤ technical language and modelling used by NICE, which are difficult to engage with or challenge

➤ concern that the NICE process doesn't take account of wider societal costs

➤ concerns about the time taken to produce guidance (reflecting concerns about delays but also potentially adverse impacts of speeding up the process)

➤ NICE 'blight' (commissioners refusing to fund technologies that have not yet been considered by NICE)

➤ variable access to technologies even when they have been recommended by NICE – there are concerns about access related both to the 'mandatory' appraisal guidance and to the implementation of clinical guidelines, which do not have the mandatory directives.

Views of individuals directly involved in producing NICE guidance

A third source of information is available from surveys of the patients, carers and members of the public who contributed directly to the production of NICE guidance. Available surveys include the following.

➤ A survey of the patient and carer members of the first 20 guideline development groups, where interviews were carried out by an independently commissioned researcher.[4]

➤ A follow-up survey seeking the views of patient and carer members and chairs of a further 38 guideline development groups that produced clinical guidelines between 2005 and 2007. This time, views were collected using a questionnaire sent out by NICE's PPIP (report in preparation).

➤ A survey of the Interventional Procedures Advisory Committee, seeking committee members' views on the content and usefulness of responses sent to patients who have had an interventional procedure.

➤ A survey of the community (lay) members and chairs of the first seven public health programme development groups that produced guidance between October 2007 and March 2009. Their views were obtained using a semi-structured questionnaire. A report of the findings is in progress.

➤ NICE's PPIP carried out a survey of people who have attended meetings of the NICE appraisal committee as patient or carer experts (report in preparation).

CHALLENGES POSED BY NEW DEVELOPMENTS

One of the challenges for NICE is that its work programmes and processes are constantly subject to expansion and review. This in turn impacts on patient and public involvement and requires the development and integration of involvement mechanisms as existing initiatives change and as new initiatives come on stream. The following sections outline some of the changes to existing initiatives and also some of the new initiatives that have broadened opportunities for involvement or posed particular challenges for engagement.

Public health

In 2005, NICE merged with the Health Development Agency (HDA), resulting in the need to extend opportunities for patient and public involvement in NICE's clinical guidance to its new public health work programme (*see* Chapter 5). This has resulted in the widening of the nature and scope of groups registering an interest in contributing to the development of NICE guidance. In particular, there has been increased interest from and involvement of organisations representing groups protected by equalities legislation that previously did not respond to invitations to engage in the production of NICE's clinical guidance.

Single technology appraisal process

NICE technology appraisals are recommendations on the use of new and existing medicines and treatments within the NHS, such as:

➤ medicines
➤ medical devices
➤ diagnostic techniques
➤ surgical procedures
➤ health promotion activities (for example, ways of helping people with diabetes to manage their condition).

We base our recommendations on a review of clinical and economic evidence.

➤ Clinical evidence measures how well the medicine or treatment works.
➤ Economic evidence measures how well the medicine or treatment works

in relation to how much it costs the NHS – does it represent value for money?

Historically NICE has appraised single or multiple products, devices or other technologies, with one or more indications using what it calls its multiple technology appraisal process. However, with pressure on NICE to speed up its process, particularly for drugs that are new to the market, it has now introduced a parallel single technology process that considers evidence on the health effects, costs and cost effectiveness of a single intervention in comparison with current standard treatment in the NHS in England and Wales. The single technology appraisal process poses particular challenges to patient and public involvement because the technologies are often referred to NICE for appraisal soon after licensing. This means that patient organisations often have no or limited contact with patients who have experience of the technology. This makes it difficult for them to draw on knowledge of patient views to make a written submission and even less likely that they are able to identify patient experts to attend the appraisal committee meeting.

More guidance, more quickly

Both the Health Select Committee report[19] and Lord Darzi's review of the NHS[20] have requested that NICE should identify ways in which it can produce more guidance more quickly. NICE has already introduced its single technology appraisal process to deliver appraisals guidance more quickly, and its 'short guidelines' programme to develop clinical guidelines in a period of six to nine months rather than the 12–18 months taken to produce longer guidelines. Speeding up the process impacts in two main ways.

➤ Consultation periods available to consultees and stakeholders are reduced, so they have even less time to consult with their constituencies to inform their input to guidance development and response to consultations.
➤ Quicker development periods result in the need to define a more limited scope for the guidance, often resulting in the omission of some key issues that stakeholders consider important.

Public advisory body meetings

In 2008, NICE announced its intention to start holding advisory committee meetings in public – it now holds meetings of its Interventional Procedures Advisory Committee, Public Health Interventions Advisory Committee (PHIAC) and technology appraisals committees in public. Increased involvement by patients and public is dependent on their willingness to participate in yet more meetings, and their willingness to share testimony of a personal or sensitive nature. All patient experts are therefore provided with written and verbal advice about what participation in the committee meetings involves, in advance of agreeing to participate. Consent forms make it clear that a patient expert can withdraw from the process at any time if they wish. Patient and carer experts are also given the opportunity to talk to the committee chair and appraisals team in advance of the meeting to give their testimony in private rather than a public session.

Patient safety

In 2007, NICE was asked to pilot the production of guidance on patient safety. One of the topics (ventilator-associated pneumonia) posed a particular challenge to obtaining a patient perspective to inform the development of the guidance. There is a national organisation representing the interests of people affected by patient-safety incidents, as well as two groups that represent the interests of patients in critical care. Yet none of these groups felt that they had a body of patient or carer views to draw on to help inform the guidance development. However, one organisation did identify a patient who had experience of critical care and could attend the committee meeting. NICE's PPIP widened invitations to trust-patient forums, patient advice and liaison services, and overview and scrutiny committees, in the hope that some of these would be able to draw on incidents reported to them by patients that would enable them to provide an informed response. We received responses from people who had personal experience of a patient safety incident, but we were unable to obtain a more collective view of the issues facing a wider cohort of patients.

Initiatives arising from the Darzi report

Another new NICE initiative is a result of Lord Darzi's review in 2008. NICE and its PPIP have been developing opportunities and materials to enable patient organisations and individual patients and the public to further contribute to the work of NICE in the form of the Quality and Outcomes Framework, NHS Evidence, Quality Standards and the development of evaluation pathways for medical devices.

REFERENCES

1 Kelson M, Longson C, Littlejohns P. NICE does consider patient views. *BMJ.* 2009; **338:** b652.
2 Kelson M. The NICE patient involvement unit. *Evid base Healthc Publ Health.* 2005; 9: 304–7.
3 Culyer AJ. Involving stakeholders in healthcare decisions: the experience of the National Institute for Health and Clinical Excellence (NICE) in England and Wales. *Healthc Q.* 2005; 8: 56–60.
4 National Institute for Health and Clinical Excellence. *A Report on a Study to Evaluate Patient/Carer Membership of the First NICE Guideline Development Groups.* London: NIHCE; June 2004.
5 Baker R. Patient involvement in national clinical guidelines: the NICE guidelines on referral for suspected cancer. *Qual Prim Care.* 2005; 13(3): 125–9.

6 Hill S, Garattini S, van Loenhout J, *et al. Technology Appraisal Programme of the National Institute for Clinical Excellence: a review by WHO.* Geneva: World Health Organization; 2003.

7 de Joncheere K, Hill S, Klazinga N. *The Clinical Guideline Programme of the National Institute for Health and Clinical Excellence (NICE): a review by the World Health Organization.* Geneva: World Health Organization; 2006.

8 Quennell P. Getting their say, or getting their way: has participation strengthened the patient 'voice' in the National Institute for Clinical Excellence? *J Manag Med.* 2001; **15**: 202–19.

9 Quennell P. Getting a word in edgeways? Patient group participation in the appraisal process of the National Institute for Clinical Excellence. *Clinical Governance: An International Journal.* 2003; **8**(1): 39–45.

10 Duckenfield M, Rangekar D. *Patient Groups and the Drug Development Process: report for the Policy Innovation Group.* London: University College London; 2004.

11 Chalmers I. Personal views: the Alzheimer's Society, drug manufacturers, and public trust. *BMJ.* 2007; **335**: 400.

12 Mentor UK Youth Involvement Project. *Mentor UK Youth Involvement Project: project report.* London: Mentor UK Youth Involvement Project; June 2008.

13 National Institute for Health and Clinical Excellence. *Interventions in Schools to Prevent and Reduce Alcohol Use Among Children and Young People: NICE public health guidance 7.* London: NIHCE; 2007. Available at: www.nice.org.uk/nicemedia/pdf/PH007Guidance.pdf (accessed 22 September 2009).

14 National Institute for Health and Clinical Excellence. *Community-Based Interventions to Reduce Substance Misuse Among Vulnerable and Disadvantaged Children and Young People: NICE public health intervention guidance 4.* London: NIHCE; 2007. Available at: www.nice.org.uk/nicemedia/pdf/PHI004guidance.pdf (accessed 22 September 2009).

15 Ferner RE, McDowell SE. How NICE may be outflanked. *BMJ.* 2006; **332**: 1268–71.

16 Herxheimer A. Relationships between the pharmaceutical industry and patients' organisations. *BMJ.* 2003; **326**: 1208–10.

17 House of Commons Health Committee. *The Influence of the Pharmaceutical Industry: fourth report of session 2004–2005.* London: London Stationery Office; 2005.

18 Sheldon TA, Cullum N, Dawson D, *et al.* What's the evidence that NICE guidance has been implemented? Results from a national evaluation using time series analysis, audit of patients' notes, and interviews. *BMJ.* 2004; **329**: 999.

19 House of Commons Health Committee. *National Institute for Health and Clinical Excellence: first report of session 2007–2008.* London: London Stationery Office; 2008.

20 Darzi A. *High Quality Care for All: NHS next stage review final report.* Cm. 7432. London: Department of Health; 2008.

CHAPTER 3

Patient and carer involvement in NICE clinical guidelines

Victoria Thomas

NICE CLINICAL GUIDELINES

NICE clinical guidelines advise health professionals, patients and carers on the best treatment and care that should be offered to people with a particular disease or condition. The guidelines are developed using a systematic methodology. The recommendations they make are based on the best available evidence, or, where evidence is lacking, on the consensus of the expert multidisciplinary groups set up to develop the guidelines.[1]

These Guideline Development Groups (GDGs) are convened by one of four National Collaborating Centres (NCCs) that NICE commissions to develop the guidelines on its behalf. Each of these centres specialises in a particular area of healthcare: mental health; cancer; acute and chronic conditions; and women's and children's health.

The GDGs are specifically convened to produce a guideline on one particular topic. Each GDG comprises healthcare professionals, researchers, and patients and carers – at least two lay members are recruited to each group (*see* 'Guideline Development Groups' below).

It should be noted that the terms 'patients and carers' are used here in their most generic sense. NICE involves a wide range of lay participants who would not choose to describe themselves as patients or carers. The terminology 'patients and carers' is used here as short-hand to include people who would call themselves, for example, service users, consumers, clients, or even, in the case of the children's or maternity topics, simply 'parents' or 'women'.

The short clinical guideline programme

NICE also has a 'short' clinical guideline development programme, which develops guideline recommendations on a discrete area of care over a much shorter period of time. These guidelines are developed in-house rather than by one of the NCCs, yet still incorporate the methodology, principles and practices of lay involvement adopted by the main guidelines programme.

How are guidelines produced

The GDGs meet regularly, over the course of about 18 months (six to nine months for the short guideline programme), and assess all the available research on one specific condition, symptom or disease. The GDGs are encouraged to actively search for qualitative research on patients' views and experiences, as well as quantitative research on the effectiveness of treatments. The findings are used to develop recommendations on how people with the condition should be treated and cared for, and to describe the evidence behind the recommendations.

Both the recommendations and the underlying evidence are subject to widespread consultation with a number of organisations that represent the interests of health professionals, commercial organisations, the NHS, and patients and carers. Any comments are considered and responded to and the guideline's recommendations are amended where necessary. The final recommendations are then published and disseminated in a number of formats, which include:

➤ the 'full guideline' that contains the guideline recommendations, details of how they were developed, and information about the evidence on which they were based
➤ a short version called the 'NICE guideline' that lists all of the guideline's recommendations (this version is not produced for the short guidelines programme)
➤ a 'quick reference guide' which is a summary of the main recommendations in the guideline and is designed to be easily accessible for health professionals
➤ an 'understanding NICE guidance' version that explains the guideline's recommendations in a more accessible way for patients, carers and members of the public.

WHY DOES NICE INVOLVE PATIENTS AND CARERS IN DEVELOPING ITS CLINICAL GUIDELINES?

NICE believes it is important to involve patients and carers in the process of making decisions about their healthcare. Patients and carers can help those responsible for developing a clinical guideline to understand what it is like to live with a medical condition or disability, and what different forms of treatment and care mean to them. For example, patients and carers can offer their insight into the practical, physical and emotional aspects of living with, or supporting someone, with a particular medical condition. This can include information about what patients want from their treatment and care, the acceptability of different treatments and their preferences for different treatment options. It can also include different views or needs for different groups of patients, for example groups differentiated by age, ethnicity, gender or disability.

WHAT SUPPORT IS AVAILABLE TO PATIENT AND CARER GUIDELINE DEVELOPMENT GROUP MEMBERS?

NICE has a team called the Patient and Public Involvement Programme (PPIP), which offers advice and support to the individual patients and carers, and their representative organisations taking part in NICE's work. The PPIP provides advice on:

➤ the guideline development process and the opportunities for patients and carers to get involved
➤ information and support at each stage of the guideline development process
➤ training for patient and carer members of individual guideline development groups.

See Chapter 2 for more information on the PPIP.

HOW NICE INVOLVES PATIENTS AND CARERS IN DEVELOPING CLINICAL GUIDELINES

Patients and carers, and the organisations that represent their interests, have the opportunity to be involved at all stages of the guideline development process, from suggesting topics for NICE to work on, through to supporting the implementation of recommendations from a published guideline.

Topic selection

The choice of topics for which NICE develops clinical guidelines is determined by the Department of Health. However anyone, including individual patients, carers and the organisations that represent their interests, can suggest topics for the Department of Health to consider. Patients and carers are also involved in groups, or 'consideration panels', that NICE convenes to filter suggestions and recommend topics to the Department of Health.

Stakeholder involvement

National patient and carer organisations can register as 'stakeholders' for a particular topic. Being a stakeholder entitles them to contribute to the development process by commenting on drafts of both the scope document and the draft recommendations. When the new clinical guideline topics are announced by the Department of Health (approximately twice a year) NICE contacts all relevant organisations (including those who have been stakeholders previously), inviting them to register an interest in any new topics relevant to them. Any organisation is welcome to register as a stakeholder – they do not have to be approached by NICE first.

Commercial, NHS and voluntary organisations can register as stakeholders, as can organisations representing healthcare professionals, patients or carers. Patient and carer organisations are usually eligible to register if they have national coverage. Occasionally regional or local organisations may be able to register if there is no national organisation representing a particular specialist interest or group of people. Organisations can register an interest in a specific guideline at any time while the guideline is being developed.

Scoping

The scope of a guideline sets out what the recommendations will and will not cover. The guideline should cover the most important areas for a particular topic, but should not be too broad as this might make it impossible to produce with available time and resources. NICE and the team at the relevant NCC produce a draft scope based on the brief description of the topic from the Department of Health.

Patient and carer stakeholder organisations are encouraged to comment on the scope, in particular on the following.

➤ Does the scope take account of issues that are important to patients and carers, such as the medicines and other treatments that patients and carers think are important?
➤ Are there any groups of patients who might need particular consideration?
➤ Does the scope unfairly exclude any groups of patients (e.g. by age or their general health)?
➤ Does the scope take into account any topic-specific information and support needs that patients and carers might have?
➤ Is the wording of the scope respectful to patients and carers, and does it enable a partnership between patient/carer and clinician?

All stakeholder organisations are invited to attend a meeting. This gives them an opportunity to become familiar with the guideline development process and to take part in detailed discussions about the proposed scope. Stakeholder organisations wishing to comment formally on the scope must also submit their comments in writing. All comments will receive a formal response from the guideline developers. The initial comments and the subsequent responses are then published on the NICE website.

Guideline development groups

Each clinical guideline has a dedicated guideline development group that comprises at least two (and sometimes more) people bringing the perspectives of patients and carers. The recruitment of patient and carer GDG members is facilitated by the PPIP. Members are sought through an open application process available on the NICE website. Anyone with an interest can apply to join a guideline development group – whether or not they are associated with a particular patient/carer organisation, although all relevant patient/carer organisations are notified about any GDG vacancies. Job descriptions, person specifications and application forms are developed for all lay vacancies on GDGs.

Patient and carer applicants do not need formal educational qualifications but do need relevant skills and experience, such as:

➤ experience relevant to the guideline topic and the issues important to people with the condition – for instance, experience of the condition as a patient or carer, or as a policy officer of a relevant patient organisation
➤ an understanding of and a willingness to reflect the experiences of a wide group of people with a condition or disease (e.g. members of a patient organisation, or support or self-help group)
➤ the time and commitment to attend the meetings, do background reading and comment on draft products
➤ good communication and teamwork skills, including respect for other people's views, and the ability to listen and take part in constructive debate
➤ the ability to maintain confidentiality as required.

Applications are passed to the staff of the relevant NCC who select applicants for the group. Those chosen often have a mix of skills. For example, the NCC may choose one member with direct personal experience as a patient or carer who can bring a depth of individual experience, and another from a relevant patient organisation who can bring a breadth of experience from a wide range of patients.

No GDG member, whether lay or health professional, is recruited to represent the views of any organisation – each member is in the group as an individual. In this way, NICE tries to avoid issues of 'representativeness' and removes the burden from the lay members of feeling that they have to represent all patients' views and experiences.

Once recruited, the lay members are given a named contact within the PPIP who will support them throughout their time on the GDG through regular email and telephone conversations. They are also sent an extensive information pack, which includes information such as a glossary of terms, an example of a patient version of a published NICE guideline, useful websites and some suggested further reading.

Lay members are also offered the opportunity to attend a specifically-designed training day. This gives them the chance to meet with other lay members on different GDGs and to learn more about the methodology used to develop the guidelines, in particular critical appraisal of research and the health-economic aspects of the process. They are also given the opportunity to meet other lay people who have completed the process, to hear about their experiences, both good and bad.

Role of lay GDG members

Patient and carer GDG members are involved in the same work as other members of the GDGs but are also asked to ensure that the patient and carer perspective is considered in the group's work. For example, they may use their specific experience and expertise to help the GDG develop patient-focused clinical questions that the research might answer. They can also assess whether the GDG's draft recommendations:

- ➤ address the treatments, interventions and outcomes that are important from the perspective of patients or carers
- ➤ take patients' and carers' views and preferences into account
- ➤ address the needs of relevant groups of patients, such as people from specific ethnic or cultural groups, or different age groups
- ➤ address patients' and carers' information, education and support needs in relation to the condition
- ➤ respect patients in wording and tone.

Patient evidence

After searching through the available research for the guideline, the developers may identify gaps in the evidence. In this instance they will approach the registered stakeholder organisations to see if they have any additional evidence that might help fill these gaps. For patient and carer organisations this can include information from surveys or questionnaires that were conducted to elicit information on the impact of a condition on people's lives or their views about care and treatment. If this is not successful, the GDG may consider other ways of obtaining additional information. For example, it may be possible to collect written testimonials (patient stories) or consult patients and carers, perhaps through a survey, workshop, discussion group or interviews. Patient and carer members of the GDG may choose to help with, or take a lead on, this work.

In addition, the GDG may need to seek advice from people outside the group. For example, the group may want to know more about the experiences or concerns of specific groups of patients. Expert advisers, including patients and carers, may be invited to one or more meetings, or be asked to contribute in writing.

Consultation comments

As with the consultation on the scope, registered stakeholders are encouraged to comment on the guideline's draft recommendations. Patient and carer stakeholder organisations are encouraged to comment on issues such as whether:

➤ the recommendations reflect what the evidence says
➤ any important evidence has not been taken into account
➤ the treatment recommended in the guideline will be acceptable to patients and carers
➤ the recommendations demonstrate the need to take into account patients' preferences – for example where the evidence suggests that two treatments are equally effective
➤ the recommendations consider the specific needs of different groups of patients, where appropriate (such as children or young people, people from specific ethnic or cultural groups)
➤ the wording used for the recommendations is clear and respectful to patients, reflecting the importance of a partnership between clinicians and patients.

The guideline developers respond to all comments from stakeholders. The comments and the formal responses to these comments are published on the NICE website at the same time as the guideline.

UNDERSTANDING NICE GUIDANCE

The recommendations in NICE clinical guidelines are translated into plain English in a version called *Understanding NICE Guidance*. This clearly sets out what the evidence indicates is the best treatment for people with a particular condition. This version is dissimilar to traditional patient information because it does not give a lot of detail about the condition itself, but rather sets out what treatment and care patients and their carers can expect from the NHS, and from their health professionals.

Its role is also to act as an aid for shared decision making between healthcare professionals and patients, as part of a clinical consultation. As it does not go into detail about the condition, this version provides details of further sources of potential support. These include key patient organisations, how patients can contact their local patient advice and liaison service, and links to statutory sources of support.

Patient and carer members of GDGs are actively involved in the development of these lay versions of the guideline, working in partnership with the NICE editorial team and the PPIP. Patient and carer members advise on the structure and content – and whether the information is right for the audience.

Implementation

Following the publication of the guideline, patient and carer organisations are encouraged to use their networks and influence to publicise the standards of care recommended in NICE guidelines. They are also asked to support their implementation both locally and nationally. NHS organisations are expected to follow recommendations in NICE clinical guidelines. This involves looking at their existing practice and making changes where needed.

Increasingly patients and carers, and the local and national organisations that represent them, are helping to support the dissemination and implementation of NICE guidelines. Examples include:

➤ publicising the guideline on their website and in mailings to members
➤ including key messages from a NICE guideline in leaflets and other materials for patients and carers
➤ conducting surveys to find out if NICE guidelines are being followed and using the findings to campaign for improvements
➤ working with NHS organisations, healthcare professionals and other patients to help put NICE recommendations into practice at a local level.

2004 REPORT

In 2004, the Patient Involvement Unit (the former name of the Patient and Public Involvement Programme), commissioned a small qualitative evaluation of the patient/carer members and chairs of NICE's first 20 GDGs. This evaluation made a number of recommendations to improve both the experience and effectiveness of having patients and carers as members of guideline development groups, many of which have been incorporated into the standard processes described above. These included:

➤ recruitment and training to follow formal and systematic processes
➤ additional information on the support available to patient/carer members
➤ selecting GDG chairs on the basis of their facilitation skills as well as clinical expertise
➤ all GDG members working to the agreed scope
➤ additional support in understanding complex scientific/technical issues
➤ a more systematic policy on making consensus recommendations.

In 2008, I conducted a survey of 126 patients, carers and chairs from GDGs to examine any outstanding issues from the recommendations from the 2004 report. The report of this survey is in preparation.

REFERENCE

1 National Institute for Health and Clinical Excellence. *The Guidelines Manual 2009.* London: NIHCE; 2009. Available at: www.nice.org.uk/aboutnice/howwework/developing niceclinicalguidelines/clinicalguidelinedevelopmentmethods/GuidelinesManua12009. jsp (accessed 22 September 2009).

CHAPTER 4

Patient involvement in NICE technology appraisals

Lizzie Amis

WHAT IS A NICE TECHNOLOGY APPRAISAL?

NICE provides guidance to the NHS on the use of selected new and existing health technologies. Health technologies are any medical interventions, such as drugs, medical devices, diagnostic techniques, surgical procedures and health promotion activities.

The process of producing this guidance is called a technology appraisal, and there are two types: single technology appraisals (STAs) and multiple technology appraisals (MTAs). The stages of these two processes are broadly similar, and I will describe them in this chapter.

STAs produce guidance on only a single technology and for only a single way that the technology is used (if it can be used in different ways or for different diseases). This means these topics have only a small amount of evidence to consider and can be done relatively quickly. MTAs however, need to consider evidence on more than one technology and/or more than one way that the technology or technologies can be used as part of one large topic. Examples include three different drugs that can all be used to treat the same group of patients or a procedure that can be used at both the early and advanced stages of a disease.

HOW NICE INVOLVES PATIENTS AND CARERS IN ITS TECHNOLOGY APPRAISALS

NICE believes it is important to involve patients and carers in producing all types of NICE guidance. Patients and carers, and the organisations that represent their interests, can be involved at all stages of the technology appraisals process, from suggesting the topics for NICE to produce guidance on, through to supporting the implementation of published guidance.

Figure 4.1 summarises the stages of a technology appraisal. The stages that have a significant level of patient public involvement are shaded.

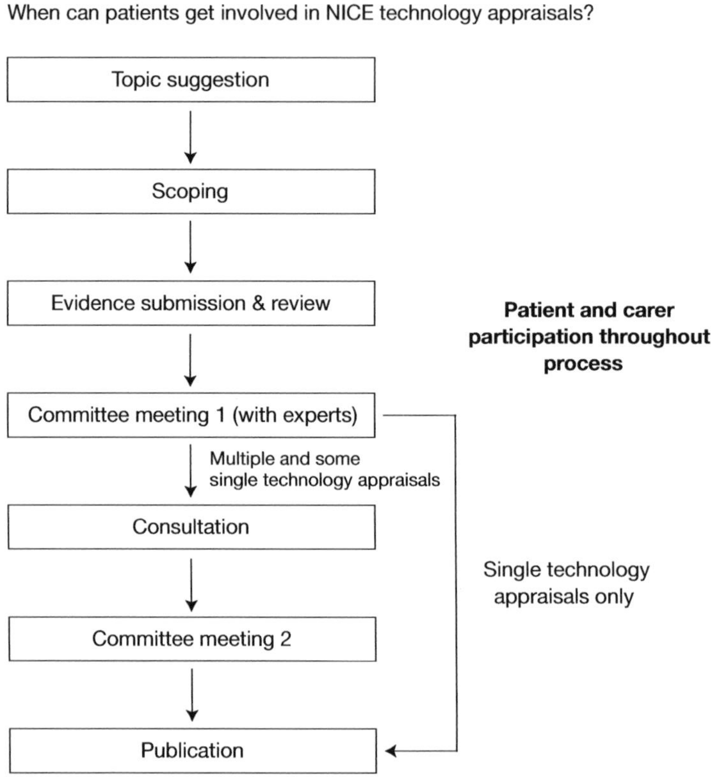

When can patients get involved in NICE technology appraisals?

FIGURE 4.1: Flow chart of the technology appraisal process (overview).

TOPIC SUGGESTION

Patients, carers and the organisations that represent their interests can suggest topics that they think NICE should develop guidance on. Suggested topics are first assessed and filtered by committees at NICE called 'consideration panels'. Each consideration panel has three lay members on it, who may be patients, carers or people from a patient organisation. The panels review evidence for each topic, including questionnaires completed by relevant patient organisations.

The Department of Health makes the final decision about which topics will go forward and be developed into guidance, taking NICE's recommendations into account.

SCOPING

The Department of Health refers topics to NICE at two separate points in the technology appraisals process. The first time the topics are referred, they are known as 'minded referrals'. The second time, after a topic has been through the technology appraisal scoping process, the topics are said to be 'formally referred'. The design of the scoping process allows each topic to be fully investigated before it starts as a full guidance topic. This ensures that the question being asked is the most appropriate for the NHS and for patients and carers.

The scoping process has two main stages – the written consultation and the workshop.

Written consultation

NICE develops two documents for consultation: the draft scope and the provisional matrix. The draft scope sets out the question that the guidance will answer. It includes which technologies will be assessed and which technologies they will be compared against ('comparator technologies'). The draft scope also covers the group of patients whose care will be covered by the guidance, such as only adult women or people with a severe form of a particular condition. It also lists the main 'outcomes' or aspects of the evidence that the assessment will use to measure how well the technologies work and whether they are value for money. Some common outcomes are: quality of life; side effects (including pain); length of life; time until the disease comes back; and other outcomes specific to certain diseases.

The provisional matrix lists all the relevant organisations that will be invited to participate in the topic as formal stakeholders. The matrix is split into two types of organisations: consultees and commentators. Consultee groups include: the manufacturer/sponsor of each of the technologies being assessed; national patient/carer organisations; and healthcare professional groups. Commentators include: relevant research groups; the manufacturer/sponsor of each of the comparator technologies; the independent academic group working with NICE on the topic; and other groups who would have a general interest in the topic. Both sets of organisations can comment in full on all consultations, but consultees can additionally submit evidence for review, nominate expert witnesses to attend the first committee meeting (except manufacturers), and can formally appeal against NICE's final guidance. I will explain these three stages more fully later in this chapter.

Both the draft scope and the provisional matrix are sent to all the groups listed on the provisional matrix for a four-week written consultation. It is important that patient/carer organisations comment on whether all the appropriate and relevant patient/carer organisations are listed, including equalities organisations, and whether the suggested outcomes and population are relevant to patients with that condition.

Workshop

All groups on the provisional matrix are invited to attend a one- to two-hour scoping workshop. The purpose of the workshop is to finalise the draft scope and provisional matrix and for all groups to reach consensus on the precise wording and content of the two documents. The comments received during the written consultation form the basis for the discussions at the scoping workshop. It is really important that groups representing patients and carers attend the scoping workshop, even if they have not sent in written comments, to ensure that all opinions and points of view are taken into account when the documents are finalised. Having the views of patients and carers represented at this stage ensures the guidance will best reflect what is important to patients and carers, and ensure the guidance is patient centred.

After the workshop, the NICE team finalises the two documents and writes a report. This report goes to the Department of Health and includes a recommendation about whether the topic is appropriate for a formal referral, and if so, when it would be most appropriate for that topic to start. At this stage there is no guarantee that a topic will go ahead. The Department of Health considers the report and informs NICE of its decision by sending through a formal final referral. It is at this point that the main section of the technology appraisal process starts: the assessment phase.

EVIDENCE SUBMISSION AND REVIEW – THE ASSESSMENT PHASE

When development for a guideline starts, NICE publishes a web page for that topic on the NICE website and this details the timetable for the different stages of the process. NICE reviews the draft scope and provisional matrix to ensure they are up to date and finalises them as the final scope and final matrix. It then sends a letter to all organisations on the final matrix, including all the patient, carer and voluntary groups, inviting them to participate in the topic. Organisations that decide to accept and participate must sign a confidentiality agreement form. The next stages of the topic are then evidence submission and nominating experts.

Evidence submission

All consultee organisations are invited to submit evidence to NICE and this is reviewed by an appraisal committee. It is important for patient and carer organisations to give a balanced view of the technologies being assessed and to give their views on questions such as:
➤ what is it like to have the condition?
➤ what are the outcomes that matter most to patients?
➤ what difference does the technology make?
➤ what it is like to use the technology and are there any costs associated with

doing so, such as having to pay transport costs because the technology can only be given in a hospital?

Patient evidence is a really important part of the evidence that is collected. Patients and carers, and the groups that represent them, have a unique insight into what it is really like to have a disease or condition and what impact the technology has on their symptoms, quality of life, and friends and family.

Nominating experts

All patient/carer organisations and healthcare professional groups are invited to nominate individuals to attend the first appraisal committee meeting as expert witnesses. Each topic normally has four experts – two clinical experts and two patient experts. Patient experts are not representatives of an organisation, despite being nominated by a consultee patient/carer group. Instead, patient experts are there to answer questions, talk about their own experience and raise issues of concern to them in the committee discussion. Patient experts can be individual patients or carers, volunteers or employees of a patient/carer or voluntary organisation, or a combination of any of those. Having experience of the condition, and ideally also the specific technology being looked at, is really important.

Patient experts are asked to sign a confidentiality agreement prior to the committee meeting and to give their consent to discussing the topic in a public session. If a patient expert would like to discuss matters that are sensitive or confidential, arrangements will be made for them to discuss these in a closed session. Each expert also sends a written personal statement that forms part of the evidence reviewed by the appraisal committee.

APPRAISAL COMMITTEE MEETINGS

The appraisal committee is an independent standing committee at NICE and has about 30 members. The committee membership reflects all groups with an interest in NICE guidance including: clinicians; NHS managers; commissioners; representatives of the pharmaceutical and medical devices industries; statisticians; and health economists. Each technology appraisal committee also has three lay members. Currently NICE has four appraisal committees that meet once a month. Technology appraisal topics cover all clinical areas from diabetes to lung cancer and from childhood asthma to schizophrenia. The appraisal committees review technologies across this range.

Committee meetings – held in public

All of NICE's standing advisory committees, including the technology appraisal committees, hold their meetings in public as part of NICE's commitment to openness and transparency. There is potential for up to 20 people to observe each meeting, including interested members of the public, members of the press and people from stakeholder organisations. The meetings are held in two parts – part one is open to the public and part two is closed to protect sensitive and confidential information.

The first appraisal committee meeting

Once all the evidence has been reviewed, it is sent to all the attendees of the first appraisal committee meeting, including the patient experts. Each topic has two committee members assigned to it as the 'lead team'; one member focuses on 'clinical effectiveness' (how well the technology works) and the other member focuses on 'cost effectiveness' (whether the technology is good value for money for the NHS). The lead team is advised by one of the lay members, who takes key responsibility for ensuring patient and public issues raised in the evidence are made explicit in the lead team's contribution.

The lead team introduces the topic at the beginning of part one of the committee meeting, and presents a summary of some of the important issues that are likely to be discussed. The presentations are followed by a full discussion in which committee members engage with the expert panel and ask them questions to help clarify the evidence and issues being discussed. Once the committee has reached the point at which they need to discuss confidential data or sensitive issues, or if they are ready to make a decision, the Chair will call an end to part one of the meeting. At this point the public observers leave the meeting. The experts normally leave at this point too, unless a patient expert wishes to discuss matters that are personally sensitive without the public gallery present, or if the Chair asks the experts to comment on confidential data.

Part two of the meeting is kept as short as it can be, to ensure the public observers will have witnessed as much as possible. The committee finish their deliberations and make their decision. For technology appraisals the decision has to be made in closed session as the implications of the decision can affect the manufacturers' share price. NICE therefore has to ensure that all interested parties are told the decision at the same time.

CONSULTATION

NICE reports the committee's decision as a formal document after the first committee meeting. For all MTA topics and most STA topics, this document is considered draft guidance and is sent out for consultation. This document is called the 'appraisal consultation document'. The document is initially sent to all consultee and commentator organisations in confidence, along with all the evidence that the committee used to make its decision. NICE places the appraisal consultation document and background evidence on its website one week later for a full public consultation and anyone with an interest can comment. The consultation closes after a further three weeks, so the consultees and commentators have four weeks in total.

For the consultation on the draft guidance, it is most important for patients, carers and the organisations that represent them to comment on whether they:

➤ agree with the provisional recommendations – and if not, why they think the committee has reached an inappropriate or incorrect decision, particularly in light of what the document says about how the committee considered the evidence and reached its decision

➤ think that the committee has failed to take account of some of the evidence, and if so, what that additional evidence is.

As shown in Figure 4.1, for some STA topics this stage does not happen – although this is only if the committee has recommended that the single technology under review can be used completely in line with the licence for that technology, with no restrictions. In this situation the committee's decision is written by NICE as final guidance; there is no consultation on this and the committee does not have a second meeting for the topic.

The second appraisal committee meeting

Following the consultation, all the comments are collated and sent to the committee in advance of their second meeting for that topic. Experts are not normally invited back for this meeting, but part one of the meeting is held in public as for the first committee meeting. The committee reviews its draft recommendations in light of the comments received, and in part two makes any changes that may be needed before deciding on their final recommendations. After the meeting, NICE writes these recommendations into the final guidance in a formal document called a 'final appraisal determination'.

Appeal

The final appraisal determination is sent to all consultee and commentator organisations. Commentators receive it for information, but consultees, including patient/carer organisations, have the right to appeal against the final guidance. There are three grounds on which consultees can appeal, as follows:

➤ if NICE hasn't followed its own predetermined process

➤ if the decision is illogical in light of the evidence it was based on

➤ if NICE has exceeded its powers, for example, the guidance will affect someone's human rights.

If no appeals are received then the final appraisal determination is published as formal NICE guidance. If one or more valid appeals are received, NICE will hold a public appeal hearing. The appeal is heard by a panel made up of non-executive members of the NICE Board, a lay member, and a representative of the pharmaceutical or medical devices industry. A lawyer is also present. The appellants set out their case and representatives of the technology appraisal committee and NICE staff who worked on the topic are present to answer the appellants' claims. If the appeal is upheld then the topic normally goes back to another committee meeting so some of the evidence, or relevant new evidence, can be reconsidered. If the appeal is dismissed then the topic proceeds to publication.

PUBLICATION
Technology appraisal guidance is published in different formats.

- The 'full guidance' contains the recommendations, details of how the decisions were reached and information about the evidence on which they were based.
- A 'quick reference guide' is a summary of the main recommendations in the full guidance and is designed to be easily accessible for health professionals.
- *Understanding NICE Guidance* explains the guidance in a way that is understandable to patients, carers and members of the public.

The *Understanding NICE Guidance* version clearly sets out how the technologies should be used in the NHS and therefore whether patients and carers should be able to access those technologies as part of their care. Its role is to act as an aid for shared decision making between healthcare professionals and patients, as part of a clinical consultation. This version also includes details of further sources of potential support, such as key patient organisations, how patients can contact their local Patient Advice and Liaison Service, and links to statutory sources of support.

HOW PATIENT AND PUBLIC INVOLVEMENT ADDS VALUE TO NICE'S TECHNOLOGY APPRAISALS GUIDANCE
NICE believes that it is very important to involve patients and carers in every technology appraisal topic. This ensures that the guidance will be patient centred and reflect the issues, concerns and views of patients and carers. In this way NICE guidance helps patients receive the best care, including access to the best drugs and technologies, whilst ensuring that the NHS spends its money wisely.

Patients, carers and groups that represent them have improved the guidance by making valuable contributions to NICE's technology appraisal topics and decision making. Some notable examples include the following.

Psoriasis

Clinical research indicated that the extent of the skin condition, psoriasis, was what most affected patients' quality of life. Patients, however, challenged this view and said that the location of the flare-up (e.g. on the face or joints) was more significant.

Kidney dialysis

When considering the topic of kidney dialysis, the committee assumed patients would prefer dialysis at home as it would be more convenient and they wouldn't have to spend money travelling to hospital. However, some patients said that they disliked home machines as it meant their illness dominated their lives.

Targeted biological therapies

Some topics have looked at a specific group of new drugs that can all be used for the same condition and are therefore alternatives to each other. The drugs have different prices and have been used in different clinical trials and so have differ-ent evidence for the committee to consider, but they also differ by how people take the drugs. Within a group of targeted biological therapies one therapy was available only at hospital through a drip (intravenously), whereas others could be taken at home as injections that the patient or a carer could administer. When patients commented on this, they said that some patients prefer self-injecting at home as it gives greater flexibility and they didn't have to pay to go to hospital. However, some patients prefer intravenous infusions as they then have fixed regular appointments; they don't have to, or are unable to, self-inject; and some people have had problems with 'sharps' collections (people coming to collect the used self-injection needles).

Age-related macular degeneration (AMD)

For AMD, a big issue was about the difference between seeing with only one eye or with two eyes. The evidence suggested that loss of sight in one eye doesn't affect quality of life very much. However, patient organisations, patients and carers disagreed and clearly indicated that there were significant negative effects on daily activities and quality of life.

Diabetes – insulin pumps

Insulin pumps allow diabetics better control of their condition. This is because the device constantly monitors the blood sugar and makes frequent small adjust-ments to the insulin needed so people don't have to rely on insulin injections that are given less frequently. Insulin pumps can be used by adults or children with diabetes, but there isn't much published evidence on how well they work in children. One of the patient experts at the committee meeting was the mother of a child who used an insulin pump and she worked with a childhood diabetes charity. She gave the committee an insight into the impact that this device has on children and how it can revolutionise their care and quality of life. This helped the committee make their decision about the usefulness of insulin pumps for children despite the lack of published evidence.

CHAPTER 5

From patient involvement in clinical guidance to lay involvement in public health guidance

Jane Cowl

In April 2005, NICE merged with the Health Development Agency and took on a new responsibility for producing public health guidance. The guidance would promote good health, prevent ill health and reduce health inequalities. As a result of this expanded remit, NICE started to develop support for involving the public – be they citizens, client groups or communities – in this new and exciting area of activity.

    This chapter describes how NICE has involved the public (both individuals and organisations representing their interests) in our public health programme, and some specific challenges that we faced. It concludes with our plans for evaluation.

APPLYING THE PRINCIPLES OF PATIENT AND PUBLIC INVOLVEMENT

In line with our commitment to 'patient-centred' clinical guidance,[1] NICE aims to produce public health guidance that takes full account of the issues that are important to the client group or target population.[2] It also aims to develop recommendations that promote partnership with, and respect for, individuals and communities. To help meet this commitment, guidance developers search for and include evidence on the views and experiences of the client group or community. NICE's Patient and Public Involvement Programme (PPIP) supports individuals and organisations that bring community perspectives (also referred to as 'lay' perspectives) to the guidance development process.

WHAT ARE LAY PERSPECTIVES IN PUBLIC HEALTH GUIDANCE?

Lay perspectives and interests on public health topics can be broader and more complex than on clinical care. Some of NICE's public health guidance may highlight potentially conflicting interests between the client group and the wider public. For example if an employer gives smokers time off to attend a smoking cessation service, non-smokers in the workforce may object. NICE's recommendation for employers to collaborate with staff and their representatives in developing a smoking cessation policy may help address such potential conflicts.[3]

When it comes to mandatory public health measures such as banning smoking in public places or compulsory wearing of seat belts in cars, there is an observable conflict between the wider public benefit and an individual's choice and freedom.

NICE asked its Citizens Council to consider whether it is legitimate for authorities to intervene in a mandatory way to address a public health problem.[4] Although the Council took the view that where possible people should have freedom of choice and be responsible for their own health, they also concluded that, when necessary, NICE should recommend mandatory interventions. The Council's deliberations informed NICE's *Social Value Judgements* paper, which sets out principles for the development of NICE guidance.[5]

Community or client perspectives are likely to differ from those of practitioners or researchers, with respect to their perceptions of the advantages and disadvantages of specific interventions or approaches. Indeed an intervention may have adverse consequences that professionals are not aware of. For example, a smoker who doesn't feel able to quit could stop seeking health advice from their GP to avoid discussions on stopping smoking.

The client group will have views on the outcomes that are important to them in relation to specific public health interventions. For example, what outcomes are important for people who want to quit smoking? An important outcome for some people may be not putting on excessive weight as a result of quitting. For others it might be the importance of maintaining a social life after quitting when most of their friends still smoke. It is essential to know what outcomes are important to the smokers themselves in order to assess if a specific approach or service is likely to be effective.

There will be a variety of needs and preferences within the client group that we need to know about as they will impact on how appropriate and acceptable specific interventions or approaches will be.

CASE STUDY: Looked after children

In 2008, we started work on a new guidance project to promote the health and well-being of children and young people in public care ('looked after children'). This was a joint guidance project between NICE and the Social Care Institute for Excellence (SCIE). Both organisations agreed on the importance of including the perspectives of children and young people in care:

- to identify their experiences, needs and views so that they could be incorporated into the guidance
- to identify desirable outcomes for interventions and protocols to support the health and well-being of this group
- to ensure, as far as possible, that interventions were accessible and acceptable to the children and young people
- to ensure the guidance maximised the ability of children/young people to participate in making decisions and choices about their lives.[6]

Although the intended beneficiaries of this guidance seemed to be a well-defined population group, there was great diversity within it. Children and young people had followed different pathways into care, and had a wide range of different needs in relation to their emotional and physical health and well-being. We had the challenge of reflecting this diversity in the guidance, bearing in mind that relevant evidence from the literature was likely to be sparse (and not up to date). In light of this, we directly consulted a diverse range of children and young people in care to help develop the guidance.

We also successfully recruited adults who had been through the public care system, to the independent advisory group for the NICE/SCIE guidance, as 'community members'.

WHO TO INVOLVE?

One particular challenge for involving the community in public health guidance is that the lay audience is much broader and less easily defined for public health than it is for clinical topics. For the latter, the focus is normally a relatively easily defined group of patients, service users and, where relevant, carers as well as the organisations that represent their interests. The following examples of public health guidance illustrate the breadth of lay audiences that we seek to involve at an individual and organisational level.

➤ For some public health topics, the potential beneficiaries may include the majority of the population. For example, NICE has published guidance on creating environments that encourage physical activity and is currently developing guidance on the prevention of cardiovascular disease. The latter guidance project is looking at population-wide activities and approaches, including mass-media health promotion campaigns, and policies related to the environment, fiscal measures and legislation.

➤ A second category of public health guidance potentially benefits a large and diverse subsection of the population, for example guidance (in development) that aims to reduce differences in the uptake of immunisation among children and young people.

➤ A third category of guidance projects focuses on a more easily defined population group yet the views of the wider community may also be relevant. For example, guidance on needle and syringe programmes is targeted at injecting drug users. Although this client group is relatively defined, the views and experiences of the wider community are also relevant because needle and syringe programmes need to operate successfully within community settings.

Identifying organisations that represent lay interests for a specific public health guidance topic

National voluntary and Non-Governmental Organisations (NGOs) and Local Involvement Networks (LINks) can register as stakeholders for individual topics of public health guidance. Once registered, NICE automatically invites them to contribute at various stages of the guidance development process.

For each new guidance topic, we consider the relevant client or population groups and with the PPIP's help, systematically seek to identify organisations that most directly represent the interests of these groups. We then invite each to participate. We personally follow up key organisations that are new or not familiar with NICE's work in order to encourage and support their involvement. Such personal contact has often proved fruitful in securing the participation of organisations that would otherwise not have become involved.

For some public health topics, we face challenges in defining lay participants and audiences. The following case study illustrates this.

CASE STUDY: Workplace smoking

When developing guidance on supporting people in the workplace who want to quit smoking (referred to here as 'workplace smoking'), we identified the following types of 'lay' organisations that could have a potential interest in the guidance:

- anti- and pro-smoking campaign groups
- groups representing patients with smoking-related conditions
- trade unions
- NGOs promoting the health of specific population groups
- NGOs providing stop-smoking services
- employers' organisations.

All these different types of organisations could be considered 'lay' organisations, but some were closer to promoting the interests of the client group (employees who smoke) than others. The following voluntary and NGOs responded and became registered stakeholders:

- Action on Smoking and Health
- Age Concern
- ASLEF (trade union for train drivers)
- Asthma UK
- Bangladeshi Stop Tobacco Project
- Breakthrough Breast Cancer
- British Ethnic Health Awareness Foundation
- British Heart Foundation
- British Lung Foundation
- Cancer Research UK
- Communication Workers Union
- Community Action Network – Health/Sport
- Confederation of British Industry
- Diabetes UK
- Disability Rights Commission
- DrugScope
- Equal Opportunities Commission
- Equalities National Council
- Fibroid Network Charity
- General Federation of Trade Unions
- GMB (general trade union)
- GMFA (gay men's health charity)
- In-Volve (works with communities on tackling drugs, crime and diversity issues)
- National Association of Head Teachers
- National Osteoporosis Society
- Public and Commercial Services Union
- QUIT (provides stop-smoking services)
- Rethink (mental health charity)
- Roy Castle Lung Foundation
- The Mentor Foundation (works with vulnerable young people)
- The Stroke Association
- Trade Union Congress
- Turning Point (works with drug users and others with complex needs)
- UNISON (public sector trade union)

As anticipated, a range of patient groups that had previously engaged with NICE on clinical topics registered for this public health guidance project, as did NGOs that supported smoking cessation. Some 'equalities' organisations that represent the interests of specific population groups also registered as stakeholders.

We find that there generally seems to be more interest from equalities groups in NICE public health topics (with their explicit remit for reducing health inequalities) than in clinical topics.

Perhaps because of NICE's reputation for clinical guidance, it has taken us longer to engage stakeholders from non-health settings, such as education and the workplace. For 'workplace-smoking' guidance, this slower engagement was evident in the case of organisations representing the interests of employers and employees. However, by the time the guidance was published in April 2007, a number of trade unions had registered as stakeholders, and three of the big unions and a key employers' organisation had contributed comments during the consultation on the draft guidance.

Identifying individuals to contribute lay perspectives to the development of public health guidance

NICE guidance is developed by independent advisory committees or groups that consider the evidence and develop recommendations. Every NICE committee and group has at least two lay/community members. To date, the minimum number for public health work has been three members and the maximum six out of a total group membership ranging from about 15 to 25. The positions are advertised on our website and through stakeholder networks. Lay/community experts may also be invited to meetings to help committees understand more about the experiences of the client groups. They may join the group as 'co-optees' to work alongside the other members (*see* below), or be invited to a specific meeting to give testimony as 'experts'.

Defining lay/community members is relatively straightforward when recruiting to advisory groups that address clinical topics because members are usually people who are patients with the condition, carers of people with the condition or members of patient groups that represent the interests of patients or carers. Defining lay/community members for public health guidance is more complicated as they are sourced from a wider range of organisations, including some that may be considered more professional than client oriented. As a result, we define lay/community members by the fact that they meet the criteria in the role description and person specification, rather than try to differentiate between the backgrounds, experience and job status of individuals.

Usually, lay or community members of NICE advisory bodies for public health topics are:

➤ community representatives and members of the client group or target population for the guidance

➤ people from voluntary, community and NGOs that are run by, or directly reflect the perspectives of client groups targeted by public health programmes and interventions.[7]

We follow the same principles as for other NICE advisory bodies when we recruit individual lay people to groups or committees for public health work. We use an open and transparent recruitment process with an explicit role description and person specification. Once recruited, the PPIP provides lay/community members with dedicated information, training and support.

The groups developing public health guidance include public health and other relevant professionals and researchers as well as lay/community members. All members have equal status, which reflects the relevance and importance of their different expertise and experience.

The recruitment panels select members of the group for their individual experience and expertise; they are not required to represent the views of an organisation or to be representative of a specific client or community group. 'Representativeness' is not relevant or achievable in terms of the relatively small numbers of people sitting on an advisory body; this applies equally to professionals on the group, as it does to lay or community members. We seek instead to recruit lay/community members who can draw on both their own understanding of community and equality issues as well as on the research evidence (which can be more representative), to ensure that these issues are deliberated and considered. The group as a whole is also required to address issues relating to health inequalities and diversity when considering the topic.

Examples of the types of people who are recruited as lay members are illustrated in Table 5.1.

NICE advisory bodies for public health guidance can co-opt additional people to contribute to their deliberations, or invite experts to give testimony to the committee or group. These co-optees and experts can include members

TABLE 5.1: Examples of lay/community membership for groups developing guidance.

Tuberculosis	*Smoking cessation*
(joint public health and clinical guidance on prevention and treatment of TB)	*(public health guidance)*
Four community members:	Four community members:
Policy officer from a refugee organisation	Ex-smoker and community development worker
A person with both TB and HIV+ status	
A recent immigrant with TB	Manager of lung cancer charity's community smoking-cessation programme
Policy officer from a lung disease charity	Ex-smoker and manager of charity's support services for smokers
	Ex-smoker and cardiac patient representative

of the client group and other people with expertise on issues that are important to specific communities or client groups. For example, two lay people with wide networks and knowledge of needle and syringe programmes gave testimony to the Public Health Interventions Advisory Committee. Their up-to-date contributions from a client perspective provided information that was not available in the research evidence and thereby added value to the development of the needle and syringe programme guidance.

Occasionally, if there is a lack of evidence on the views and experiences of client groups, NICE commissions primary research to gather it. An example is a project that aimed to prevent the uptake of smoking by children and young people. Contracted researchers convened focus groups with young people to find out their views and experiences. Their views were sought on new issues for which there was no research evidence, such as their use of new media and raising the legal age for buying cigarettes from age 16 to 18. Participants were recruited to achieve the required diversity in terms of age, gender and smoking status, and young people excluded from school were included. The researchers used an interactive electronic voting tool on sensitive issues.[8]

OPPORTUNITIES FOR INVOLVEMENT

This chapter has focused on the involvement of the public at the stages of scoping, developing and validating NICE guidance. However, NICE provides opportunities for members of the public (and/or organisations representing their interests) to contribute at all stages of work on public health guidance. These include:

➤ suggesting topics for NICE to develop guidance
➤ scoping each guidance topic
➤ developing the guidance (considering the evidence and developing recommendations)
➤ validating the guidance (consultation on and revision of the draft guidance)
➤ disseminating and implementing the guidance.

This is outlined in more detail in Table 5.2 opposite.

EVALUATION
Ongoing activities

In the process of supporting lay participants in NICE's public health work, the PPIP receives informal feedback on what is working well and acts on any problems that need addressing. We also seek written feedback from participants

TABLE 5.2: Opportunities for lay involvement in public health guidance.

Stage and nature of involvement	Involvement opportunities – ORGANISATIONS	Involvement opportunities – INDIVIDUALS
Topic selection		
Anyone can suggest a topic for future NICE guidance	Yes	Yes
	No	Yes
A Topic Consideration Panel, which includes three lay members, filters and prioritises suggestions for future public health guidance		
Defining the scope of each guidance topic		
NICE consults stakeholders on the draft scope that sets out what the guidance will and will not cover. Organisations representing public interests (usually national voluntary organisations or NGOs) can influence the nature and direction of the guidance by contributing comments as part of this consultation process	Yes	No
Development of guidance		
Participation through membership of independent advisory groups that consider the evidence and develop recommendations. For public health topics, there are two different types of guidance development groups:	No	Yes
	No	Yes
a standing committee called the Public Health Interventions Advisory Committee (PHIAC) that works on all intervention topics and includes four lay members		
a programme development group that is set up for each guidance programme and includes at least three lay people who bring the perspectives of the client group or community		
Co-optees and experts – PHIAC and the programme development groups co-opt additional people to contribute to their deliberations, or they invite experts to give testimony to the committee or group. This includes lay or community experts/co-optees		
Validation		
Consultation with stakeholders on the draft guidance – this is an opportunity for stakeholder organisations to raise any outstanding issues of concern from the perspective of the client group or target population for the guidance	Yes	No
	No	Yes

(continued)

Stage and nature of involvement	Involvement opportunities – ORGANISATIONS	Involvement opportunities – INDIVIDUALS
Validation (continued)		
Fieldwork – the draft recommendations are tested out with practitioners including people working for non-governmental, voluntary and community. organisations. We are also developing our approach to consulting directly with members of the client group		
Dissemination and implementation of guidance		
Lay people who have been involved in the development of public health guidance often play a role in its launch and other dissemination activities. We also encourage national and local voluntary organisations, NGOs and LINks to promote NICE guidance and use it to support their own priorities on improving health	Yes	Yes

at our training days for lay/community members of advisory groups, and this informs our regular reviews of the training programme. Informally we have received positive examples of the impact of lay/community involvement, both from lay people themselves and other group members and observers. We have started to collect examples of the impact or difference that lay/community involvement makes to public health guidance.

Formal evaluation
The PPIP is currently developing a formal evaluation process for lay/community involvement in developing public health guidance, so that we have a systematic way of learning from what works well and what needs to be improved. This summer (2009) we are evaluating lay/community involvement on the programme development groups (the independent advisory groups that NICE sets up to develop public health programme guidance). This project involves canvassing the views of former community members and chairs of the groups that have produced public health guidance to date, using a semi-structured questionnaire.

As part of this survey, we are analysing anonymous demographic information from respondents, which includes a category about the educational level of the community members. NICE routinely collects equalities monitoring data for members of its independent advisory bodies in relation to the six equalities strands of gender, race/ethnicity, disability, age, religion/faith and sexual orientation. However, as education level is very pertinent to health inequalities, we have added this dimension for the purpose of this survey. Although formal qualifications are not a requirement of lay/community membership on NICE advisory groups, successful applicants do need to have the ability to draw on the research evidence (with the help of the training and support that NICE provides). We recognise that this (and other criteria) may exclude the least advantaged in the client group or target population from participation in this type of collaborative activity, but will await the findings from the survey.

A report of this evaluation project will be produced in Autumn 2009 and we will be acting on the findings.

CONCLUSION

NICE has developed its approach to lay involvement in its public health guidance, building on the experience of patient and carer involvement in clinical guidance. This has involved addressing the greater complexity of the lay audience for public health guidance. We will continue to refine our approach in response to feedback and lessons learnt.

REFERENCES

1 National Institute for Health and Clinical Excellence. *Patient and Public Involvement Policy.* London: NIHCE. Available at: www.nice.org.uk/getinvolved/patientandpublicinvolvement/ patientandpublicinvolvementpolicy/patient_and_public_involvement_policy.jsp (accessed 22 September 2009).

2 In-Volve. *People and Participation: how to put citizens at the heart of decision making.* London: Involve; 2005.

3 National Institute for Health and Clinical Excellence. *Workplace Health Promotion: how to help employees to stop smoking: NICE public health intervention guidance 5.* London: NIHCE; 2007. Available at: www.nice.org.uk/nicemedia/pdf/PHI005guidance.pdf (accessed 22 September 2009).

4 National Institute for Health and Clinical Excellence. *NICE Citizens Council Report: mandatory public health measures.* London: NIHCE; 2005. Available at: www.nice.org. uk/nicemedia/pdf/NICE_Citizens_Council_Report_Public_Health.pdf (accessed 22 September 2009).

5 National Institute for Health and Clinical Excellence. *Social Value Judgements: principles for the development of nice guidance.* 2nd ed. London: NIHCE; 2008. Available at: www.nice. org.uk/media/C18/30/SVJ2PUBLICATION2008.pdf (accessed 22 September 2009).

6 National Institute for Health and Clinical Excellence and Social Care Institute for Excellence. *Plan for Involving Children and Young People and Their Families, and Incorporating Their Views.* Unpublished paper. 2008.

7 National Institute for Health and Clinical Excellence. *Lay Payment Policy.* Unpublished paper. 2008.

8 National Institute for Health and Clinical Excellence. *Mass-Media and Point-of-Sales Measures to Prevent the Uptake of Smoking by Children and Young People: NICE public health guidance 14.* London: NIHCE; 2008. Available at: www.nice.org.uk/nicemedia/pdf/ PH14fullguidance.pdf (accessed 22 September 2009).

CHAPTER 6

Patient involvement in NICE interventional procedures programme

Emma Chambers

The Interventional Procedures Programme was set up in 2003 to make recommendations about whether interventional procedures that are used to diagnose and treat ill health are safe and work well enough to be used routinely.

An interventional procedure can be defined as a procedure that is used for diagnosis or treatment that involves:

➤ making a cut or a hole to access the inside of a patient's body – for example, when carrying out an operation or inserting a tube into a blood vessel
➤ accessing a body cavity (such as the digestive system, lungs, womb or bladder) without cutting into the body – for example, examining or carrying out treatment on the inside of the stomach using an instrument inserted through the mouth
➤ using electromagnetic radiation (such as X-rays, lasers, gamma-rays and ultraviolet light) – for example, using a laser to treat an eye problem.

NICE assesses procedures that are new to the NHS and for which there is uncertainty about their efficacy and/or safety. NICE does not look at procedures that are already used as standard practice in the NHS as their risks and benefits are widely known.

NICE encourages individual patients, patient organisations, carers and members of the public to contribute to the development of interventional procedures guidance. They can get involved in the following ways.

➤ **Notification** – anybody can suggest a topic to be reviewed by the Interventional Procedure Programme. Suggestions for topics usually come from clinicians who wish to perform a new procedure, but they can also come from patients or patient organisations. For example, NICE was notified about the 'deep dermis injection of non-absorbable gel polymer filler (Bio Alcamid) for lipoatrophy' procedure by a patient who had undergone the procedure.

➤ **Patient commentator** – members of the public who have: undergone a procedure; are the carer of someone who has done so; or have been offered the procedure and declined it, can act as patient commentators. Patient commentators complete a questionnaire about their own personal experiences. This information helps the Interventional Procedures Advisory Committee (IPAC) take patient perspectives into account alongside the published research when developing its draft recommendations about a procedure.

➤ **Lay committee member** – the IPAC currently has two lay members who have an equal status on the group. One of their key roles is to ensure that patient and carer views and experiences inform the Committee's decisions. Lay vacancies for the IPAC are advertised when available.

➤ **Draft guidance consultee** – NICE actively encourages relevant patient/carer organisations to comment on draft guidance when it is published, and also encourages patient organisations to publicise consultations through their website/newsletters to allow individual patients the opportunity to comment.

This chapter will focus on patient commentators, lay committee members and draft guidance consultees.

OBTAINING PATIENT VIEWS TO INFORM IPAC DECISION MAKING – PATIENT COMMENTATORS

The Interventional Procedures Programme seeks the views of patients who have had experience of an interventional procedure. It asks trusts who offer the procedure to send a questionnaire to a sample of past patients. The responses to the questionnaire are used by the IPAC to inform their discussions. This information is used to give a patient-focused context to the published research. It can be particularly helpful to the Committee when there is no published research on patient views. The patient commentator process is as follows.

THE PATIENT COMMENTATOR PROCESS

- The Interventional Procedures Programme alerts the Patient and Public Involvement Programme (PPIP) that a procedure has provisionally been taken on by the programme.
- The PPIP identifies trusts that are performing the procedure.
- The PPIP contacts the Medical Director and Chief Executive of the trust to

gain consent for the project to go ahead.

- Medical Directors give consent for the project to go ahead and identify a contact person for the PPIP to liaise with.
- The provisional scope for the procedure is agreed at the IPAC meeting.
- The PPIP team contacts the identified contact person within the trust, to find out patient numbers.
- The PPIP prepares the patient packs to send to the individual patients. This includes: the questionnaire, an information sheet explaining what patients need to do, a covering letter that briefly explains why we are contacting them and a consent form that they need to sign to allow us to use the information they supply.
- Patients send their completed questionnaires direct to the PPIP.
- If more than four questionnaires are received, the PPIP will summarise all patient views in a report to be presented to the Committee. Otherwise anonymous questionnaires will be included in the Committee papers.
- Regardless of how many questionnaires are received, copies of all the anonymous patient questionnaires are sent to the two lay members of the Committee. This allows them to raise further patient issues that they feel may have been missed if a summary was produced for the Committee.

This can be a time-consuming process, and is largely dependent on response times. Once the PPIP has been notified about a procedure, the minimum amount of time that that is needed to get patient input is 10 weeks.

Patient involvement at this stage of guidance development is somewhat different to that of other programmes within NICE. This is due to the nature of interventional procedures, as they are often new and innovative procedures that have been carried out in only small numbers. Therefore individual patients are hard to locate, and it is necessary to make contact with patients through their trusts.

The number of questionnaires sent out can vary considerably, a reflection of the numbers of patients who are offered different procedures. For example, with one procedure we provided the Committee with just one questionnaire from the only patient in the UK to have had the procedure and survived. Conversely, for procedures involving a much larger number of patients, we ask trusts to send out questionnaires to 60 randomly selected patients.

We face a number of challenges when trying to find patient commentators for the Interventional Procedures Programme. The PPIP process for identifying patient commentators relies heavily on individual trusts sending out information on our behalf, often with short deadlines. As a result, it is inevitable that sometimes trusts will be unable to complete our requests within the specified timelines due to other pressures within the trust.

Our process also relies on patient compliance with regards to filling out our questionnaires. We are unable to follow up our approaches to ensure a good response rate. Data protection restrictions prohibit us from gaining individual patient data, and we do not currently ask trusts to send reminders owing to the large administrative workload. Despite this our typical response rate for returned questionnaires is 45%; but this can vary from zero to 100%.

Finally, procedures are not always suitable for patient comment. This may be because they are an intraoperative procedure that patients will not know that they are having, such as an intraoperative red blood cell salvage during radical prostatectomy. If the procedure is of a sensitive nature it would be inappropriate for NICE to contact the individual patient or carer, for example, after therapeutic hyperthermia with intracorporeal temperature monitoring for hypoxic perinatal brain injury.

USING PATIENT VIEWS TO INFORM IPAC DECISION MAKING

Patient commentator views are used by the Committee to inform the discussion about patient-related outcomes, potential side effects or quality-of-life issues.

An example of the contribution the patient commentator process can make is the 'deep dermal injection of non-absorbable gel polymer for HIV-related facial lipoatrophy' procedure. Patients who had received this filler for facial wasting commented extensively on the positive psychological impact of the treatment and many patients no longer needed counselling. Comments included:

'Hardly any psychiatric input these days (previously seen monthly)'

'My destroyed self-esteem was dramatically improved'

'Felt quite depressed before, now feel empowered'

The patient commentator responses were well received by the Committee and resulted in the following sentence being added to the draft guidance:

'The Committee noted that facial lipoatrophy is a distressing and disabling condition affecting patients with HIV, whose quality of life may be significantly improved by effective treatment of this condition. Deep dermal injection of non-absorbable gel polymer is one treatment option for these patients.'

Where patient commentator opinions are available, the interventional procedures 'overview' (the document that sets out the available evidence) will acknowledge that patient opinion was obtained.

When patient commentators have provided additional evidence to that reported in the published literature or that supplied by clinical advisors to the programme, this information will also be included in the interventional procedures overview.

Any additional safety and efficacy data identified by patient commentators will also be included in the interventional procedures consultation document, which sets out the draft recommendations.

THE CONSULTATION PROCESS

Patient organisations and individual patients also contribute to the Interventional Procedures Programme through the consultation process. For each procedure considered by the IPAC, the PPIP contacts national patient organisations that represent patients affected by the condition(s) relevant to the procedure. Patient organisations are asked if they would like to participate in the consultation process, and those that express an interest in being involved are contacted by the Interventional Procedures team who alert them that the consultation period has begun. A lay description of the procedure is included in this information to help organisations understand if/how the procedure is relevant to them. Patient organisations are also sent guidance prepared by the PPIP team on what kind of information to include in a consultation response.

The PPIP proactively seeks national patient organisation responses. It also encourages local patient organisations and individual patients to comment on the guidance if they wish to. Patient organisations are free to publicise the consultation to its members in various forms, including linking to the consultation on their website, or in newsletters.

NICE welcomes patient organisation and individual patient/carer/parent responses and advises them to share their views on:

➤ the provisional recommendations
➤ how well the procedure works, including benefits or drawbacks to the patient that may have been overlooked
➤ how safe (or unsafe) the procedure is, including any pain, side effects or complications that occurred.

The PPIP team are always available to support any patient organisation, or individual patient/carer/parent who may wish to make a consultation comment.

Any additional safety or efficacy information supplied by patients or patient organisations can directly influence the final guidance, and can result in the addition of new recommendations or changes to existing ones.

This is illustrated in the following example.

> **MAKING A DIFFERENCE AT CONSULTATION: A CASE STUDY**
> (High-dose-rate brachytherapy for cervical cancer)

The consultation on this procedure generated a total of six responses from patient organisations or individual patients who had undergone the procedure. Five of the six responses documented the fact that having the procedure was both distressing and painful.

This was an aspect of the procedure that was not identified as part of the clinical evidence nor was it commented on by any of the programme's clinical advisers. Therefore, as a direct result of patient comments at the consultation phase, the following recommendation was added to the guidance:

'Clinicians should ensure that patients have appropriate counselling and pain management. In addition, use of the Institute's Information for the public is recommended.'[1]

As with the questionnaires, response rates at the consultation phase can vary due to the very nature of interventional procedures. Some procedures that are considered will have a fairly large patient base, and the procedure will be known by patient organisations. A good example of this is the 'functional electrical stimulation for drop foot of central neurological origin' procedure. There is a large population of patients for this procedure, such as those with MS, stroke, cerebral palsy and spinal cord injuries. There are also a number of large centres across the UK who offer this procedure. As a result, not only were we able to gain patient opinion while the Committee formulated its recommendations, but we were able to publicise the consultation through patient organisation websites and newsletters, and therefore gain a large number of consultation responses.

Conversely, a number of procedures that the IP team look at are very novel and sometimes have only been performed a handful of times across the whole world. A good example of this is the 'percutaneous epicardial mapping and ablation for atrial fibrillation' procedure, as this was not being performed in the UK at the time of evaluation. In situations like this it is impossible to gain individual patient comments while the Committee is drafting its recommendations. It is often the case for novel procedures that have not yet been adopted in the UK, that patient organisations are also unable to comment on them due to a lack of knowledge/awareness.

Over the past few years patient and public involvement has evolved a lot in the Interventional Procedures Programme. We have successfully piloted and implemented the patient commentator process, and we have made significant changes to the way we invite people to participate in the consultation process. This has led to much more systematic patient and public involvement across the Interventional Procedures Programme.

These changes have not only led to more patient views and experiences being fed into the programme, but have ultimately enhanced the guidance either by supporting the available evidence and clinical specialists views, or by providing the Committee with further outcomes that has resulted in new information being introduced into the guidance.

REFERENCE

1 National Institute for Health and Clinical Excellence. *High Dose Rate Brachytherapy for Carcinoma of the Cervix: NICE interventional procedure guidance 160.* London: NIHCE; 2006. Available at: www.nice.org.uk/nicemedia/pdf/IPG160guidance.pdf (accessed 22 September 2009).

CHAPTER 7

Patient and voluntary organisation support for implementing NICE guidance

Victoria Thomas

NICE has a commitment to involve patients, carers and the public in its work and this extends beyond their involvement in NICE's decision making, and guidance development. Patients and the public also have a key role in helping to promote, disseminate and implement the guidance that NICE produces. NICE's Patient and Public Involvement Programme (PPIP) supports these individuals and organisations in their initiatives to increase awareness of NICE's recommendations for best practice.

Supporting the implementation of NICE guidance offers benefits to patients and carers. It can help them to:

➤ receive care in line with the best available evidence of clinical and cost effectiveness

➤ feel empowered and accountable for their care as they know how they will be cared for in a consistent evidence-based approach – this will build their confidence in NHS services

➤ improve their own health and prevent disease.

HOW CAN PATIENTS AND THE PUBLIC HELP PUT NICE'S GUIDANCE INTO PRACTICE?

Patients, carers and members of the public are in a unique position to identify when things are going well or badly in terms of the care they receive. By involving them in getting NICE guidance into practice, organisations can help to ensure that the recommendations from NICE are used in ways that are suitable, accessible and easily available to the people they affect.

Involving patients and the public also helps organisations to ensure openness and accountability in the process of 'implementation'. Patients and healthcare professionals may have very different views about the sort of care that is currently being provided (and whether NICE recommendations are already in place) and how best to provide or organise care in line with NICE recommendations. This could have an impact on how easy it is to put the recommendations into practice. In addition, the particular circumstances of the patients in a local area may need to be taken into account by healthcare or other organisations before any guidance is implemented. For example, the ethnic make-up or relative affluence of the local population may affect how certain recommendations are put into practice.

All NICE guidance is produced in versions written specifically for patients and members of the public. These easy-to-read versions, known as the *Understanding NICE Guidance* series, enable the public to identify if NICE's recommendations are being followed. Local and national patient, carer and voluntary organisations can also help disseminate these lay versions of NICE guidance to their members and contacts.

There are many national policies and local requirements for the NHS to involve patients and the public in its activities; helping to put NICE guidance into practice is one way that they can work toward fulfilling these requirements.

INVOLVING PATIENTS AND THE PUBLIC IN NICE'S IMPLEMENTATION ACTIVITIES

As described in previous chapters, NICE actively promotes and supports the involvement of patients, carers and the public in its guidance development work. The PPIP applies the same systematic principles of involvement and engagement to NICE's work on implementation. This is achieved in a number of ways as described below.

Fieldwork

NICE has a team of field consultants that work closely with local trusts, authorities, councils and networks to support the implementation of NICE guidance.[1] Consultants are allocated regions within England and they encourage local organisations to discuss their local patient and public involvement activities and how these are being employed to support the implementation of NICE guidance. They are supported by a number of practical documents and information developed in conjunction with the PPIP (*see* 'Supporting materials' below).

Commissioning

NICE has a team that produces 'commissioning guides' to support commissioners in primary care trusts. The team helps commissioners to calculate their local needs in terms of financial, staff and equipment resources in order to implement elements of NICE guidance.[2]

Lay members of the Commissioning Programme's Steering Group have experience of local NHS services and the commissioning process. Commissioning guides are produced in line with patient and public involvement policies. The topic-specific guides also make reference to the 'patient-centred' recommendations from the guidance on which they are based, which can include aspects such as patient choice, information and support, and informed decision making.

Implementation support

NICE has a team that works on systems to support the implementation of NICE guidance. The team gathers intelligence about uptake rates and examples of good practice relating to systems that allow easy access to information on what NICE has recommended. The team also looks at forward planning for the NHS and works with local authorities to identify publication dates for NICE guidance. The team also supports educational initiatives by the Healthcare Commission and the Department of Health.[3]

An implementation support team produces practical tools such as locally-adaptable slide sets, audit criteria and detailed implementation advice. The team works closely with national organisations and policy initiatives to ensure that the advice is appropriate to the NHS and others involved in implementing NICE guidance.[4]

The main area in which patients and the public are involved in NICE's implementation activities is in developing the support tools for trusts and local authorities. These are primarily based on NICE's clinical guidelines and public health guidance, which cover extensive pathways of care or large-scale health promotion or preventive-health activities. These types of guidance are subject to an eight-week consultation period. Organisations that represent the interests of health and public health professionals, manufacturers, patient, carer and voluntary organisations, and NHS trusts and public health service providers, comment on the draft recommendations during this time.

An implementation planning meeting is held during this consultation period. These meetings invite the key national organisations and policy-makers to discuss the draft recommendations and to consider the implications of these recommendations in relation to current practice. The organisations are also asked to describe any policy initiatives that might help or hinder the likely implementation of the recommendations. The meeting is not an opportunity for the attendees to register their comments on the draft recommendations – this must be done through the formal written submission processes.

Following this meeting, the information is collated and used as the basis to develop the implementation support tools produced in-house by NICE. Drafts of these tools are circulated to the organisations that attended the planning meetings to ensure that any concerns are incorporated and reflected.

SUPPORT ROLE OF THE PATIENT AND PUBLIC INVOLVEMENT PROGRAMME

The PPIP works closely with all strands of the implementation team at NICE and also supports the individuals and organisations that are an integral part of this work. The team provides support by recruiting the individuals who work with the implementation department of NICE, and once recruited, offers induction, ongoing support and training to help these individuals fully realise their roles in representing the interests and views of patients, carers and the public.

Supporting materials

The PPIP produces a range of materials that support the activities of both the implementation team at NICE and the patients, carers and the public who work with them. These include the following.

➤ Information about how the NHS and other organisations can harness the skills and experiences of local people to help support the implementation of NICE guidance. This is used by the implementation consultants as part of their fieldwork.[5]

➤ A slide set for locally representative organisations such as Local Involvement Networks (LINks) explains their options for involvement with NICE in both the development and implementation of its guidance. This can be used locally by trusts or LINks themselves or by PPIP staff for informing and training LINks about NICE's patient and public involvement activities.

➤ The PPIP produces information on what people can do if they feel they are eligible for treatment or interventions recommended by NICE, but these are not being offered locally.[6,7]

➤ Key patient organisations' contact details are included in the 'understanding NICE guidance' series. The PPIP contacts each of the organisations that could potentially be included to ask for their explicit permission for inclusion.

➤ The PPIP publishes a collection of activities undertaken by individual patients and members of the public and voluntary organisations that support the implementation of NICE guidance.[8]

Developing implementation support tools

The PPIP also encourages the involvement of voluntary organisations in developing the implementation support tools described above. The team has a role in determining the most appropriate voluntary organisations to be invited to the implementation planning meetings and equips them with support materials that explain the purpose of the meeting and what role patient, carer and other voluntary organisations can play. Organisations that are selected are those likely to have the most influence in promoting the guidance to their members and to the wider community.

Following the planning meeting, the PPIP contacts the relevant organisations and outlines what options are available to them if they want to help support the implementation of the guidance. They are directed to examples of initiatives and activities undertaken by other voluntary organisations and individuals, with a view that these might act as inspiration to others. They are also asked to comment on drafts of the implementation support tools to ensure that the appropriate messages are included.

LAY ACTIVITIES TO SUPPORT IMPLEMENTATION

A wide range of activities has been undertaken by patient, carer and voluntary organisations, as well as by individual patients, carers and service users to help promote NICE guidance and support its implementation. Examples of these include:

Awareness-raising campaigns

Breakthrough Breast Cancer www.breakthrough.org.uk
Based on the NICE Familial Breast Cancer guideline, Breakthrough Breast Cancer campaigns to improve the availability of breast-screening services for women at an increased risk of breast cancer due to their family history.

Promotion at national conferences

National Kidney Federation (NKF) www.kidney.org.uk
The NKF promotes many of the NICE guidelines at the NKF annual conference and at other regional and national meetings attended throughout the year. Information about NICE and its work is also included in the NKF national magazine, *Kidney Life*, and on the organisation's website. Further information, advice and help with the various NICE guidelines is available to patients and units through the NKF helpline and the NKF advocacy services.

Complementary leaflets and posters

Action on Smoking and Health (ASH) www.ash.org.uk

ASH produced guidance drafted by experts involved in the original smoking-cessation guidelines to assist health professionals prior to the publication of the NICE guidance on nicotine replacement therapy and varenicline. This highlights the key recommendations and links directly to the NICE guidance.

Surveys and audits

Multiple Sclerosis Trust www.mstrust.org.uk

The MS Trust has done a comprehensive audit of NHS services for people with MS, comparing them with recommendations in the NICE 2003 guideline. This project was conducted in association with the Royal College of Physicians and the Trust intends to run it every two years. The results of the second audit were published in July 2008 and still show significant gaps.

Direct funding to the NHS

Parkinson's Disease Society (PDS) www.parkinsons.org.uk

NICE's Parkinson's disease guideline recommends that all people with Parkinson's disease should have: their diagnosis made by a specialist; regular access to a specialist nurse; and access to therapies. The PDS has helped many local health organisations scope their Parkinson's services and can support local teams to find a model of specialist Parkinson's services that works for them. The PDS provides pump-priming funding for specialist nurses to help ensure every person with Parkinson's has the support of a key professional.

Training and support for health professionals

The Royal College of Psychiatrists www.rcpsych.ac.uk/crtu/centre
forqualityimprovement/self-harmproject.aspx

The Royal College of Psychiatrists has developed a multidisciplinary self-harm training programme with the help of service users. This programme brings together professionals from emergency departments, mental health and ambulance services to review and improve the service they provide to people who self-harm. Attendees are provided with training materials written by service users as well as information for service users, such as a list of helplines, a first aid leaflet and a list of distraction techniques.

Other general promotional activities

Gloucester Primary Care Trust **www.glospct.nhs.uk/content/news/2008/
january/news310108.html**
'Working better by working together' was a local action plan that engaged with
statutory, voluntary and community groups to help implement NICE guidance on
physical activity and environment.

The PPIP collates information about activities such as those described above
and records them on a database. This is available on the NICE website and is
regularly updated.[9] The database serves a number of purposes.
➤ It is a record of good practice in implementing NICE guidance.
➤ It promotes the added value of patient, carer and public involvement in
   supporting the implementation of the guidance.
➤ It acts as a 'menu' of examples from which other voluntary and local
   organisations can draw motivation to develop their own initiatives to
   support the implementation of guidance of interest to them and their
   members.

The examples in the database demonstrate that a diverse group of people is
involved in these activities. The greatest proportion comes from large national
organisations that represent patients', carers' and communities' interests.
However small groups, local organisations and individual service users are all
represented and in some instances, several organisations work together to support implementation. The activities described vary widely in their range and
scale.

The examples from patient, carer and voluntary organisations reveal an
interesting aspect to the work that is being undertaken to support the promotion, dissemination and implementation of NICE guidance. Rather than it being
solely the domain of health and public health professionals, commissioners
and NHS managers, it demonstrates a clear role for lay people and the organisations that represent them in helping to put NICE guidance into practice. It also
demonstrates an appetite from these organisations and individuals to support
the NHS and wider health communities in these activities, from small-scale
awareness raising to considerable financial input.

These examples sit alongside other collections of information about implementation activities. Examples of good practice implementation initiatives,
primarily from NHS trusts, are collated in a parallel database, known as the
shared-learning database.[10]

Anyone wishing to share their own work to support the implementation
of NICE guidance can submit an example. If the initiative is patient led or

undertaken by a patient or voluntary organisation, please contact the PPIP (patientandpublicinvolvement@nice.org.uk). Examples can also be submitted for the shared-learning database: www.nice.org.uk/usingguidance/sharedlearningimplementingniceguidance/submitanexample/submit_an_example.jsp

REFERENCES

1 National Institute for Health and Clinical Excellence. *The NICE Field Team.* London: NIHCE. Available at: www.nice.org.uk/usingguidance/niceimplementationprogramme/introducing_local_nice_representatives.jsp (accessed 22 September 2009).

2 National Institute for Health and Clinical Excellence. *Commissioning Guides: supporting clinical service redesign.* London: NIHCE. Available at: www.nice.org.uk/usingguidance/commissioningguides/bytopic.jsp (accessed 22 September 2009).

3 National Institute for Health and Clinical Excellence. *Using Guidance.* London: NIHCE. Available at: www.nice.org.uk/usingguidance (accessed 22 September 2009).

4 National Institute for Health and Clinical Excellence. *Implementation Tools.* London: NIHCE. Available at: www.nice.org.uk/usingguidance/implementationtools/implementation_tools.jsp (accessed 22 September 2009).

5 National Institute for Health and Clinical Excellence. *Involving Patients and the Public in Implementing NICE Guidance.* London: NIHCE. Available at: www.nice.org.uk/usingguidance/benefitsofimplementation/involving_patients_and_the_public_in_implementing_nice_guidance.jsp (accessed 22 September 2009).

6 National Institute for Health and Clinical Excellence. *Accessing Treatment Recommended by NICE in England.* London: NIHCE; 2008. Available at: www.nice.org.uk/media/654/22/AccessingTreatmentRecommendedByNICEEngland.pdf (accessed 22 September 2009).

7 National Institute for Health and Clinical Excellence. *Accessing Treatment Recommended by NICE in Wales/Cael gafael ar driniaeth a argymhellir gan NICE.* London: NIHCE; 2007. Available at: www.nice.org.uk/usingguidance/benefitsofimplementation/accessingtreatmentinwales.jsp (accessed 22 September 2009).

8 National Institute for Health and Clinical Excellence. *Patient and Public Activities to Support the Use of NICE Guidance – June 2009.* London: NIHCE; 2009. Available at: www.nice.org.uk/usingguidance/benefitsofimplementation/benefits_of_implementation.jsp?domedia=1&mid=AD865978–19B9-E0B5-D40457F95759AF2F (accessed 22 September 2009).

9 National Institute for Health and Clinical Excellence. *Putting Guidance Into Practice.* London: NIHCE. Available at: www.nice.org.uk/getinvolved/patientandpublicinvolvement/puttingguidanceintopractice.jsp (accessed 22 September 2009).

10 National Institute for Health and Clinical Excellence. *Shared Learning: implementing NICE guidance.* London: NIHCE. Available at: www.nice.org.uk/usingguidance/sharedlearning implementingniceguidance/shared_learning_implementing_nice_guidance.jsp (accessed 22 September 2009).

CHAPTER 8

Community engagement to improve health: how well is NICE implementing its own recommendations?

Laura Norburn

In February 2008, NICE published its ninth piece of public health guidance titled *Community engagement to improve health*.[1,2] The guidance aims to 'support those working with and involving communities in decisions on health improvement that affect them'. This chapter considers the work NICE is undertaking around community engagement and assesses the extent to which it is performing in line with the recommendations. This chapter will also identify three main areas for development and areas where, because NICE has a mainly national remit, some of the recommendations are incompatible.

BACKGROUND INFORMATION

The NICE community engagement guidance identifies a number of groups that should act on the recommendations, such as the NHS, local authorities and other public sector organisations, community organisations and community representatives with an interest in health. Some of the recommendations are directed at a particular group, such as commissioners and providers in public sector organisations, but most of the recommendations are directed at all the groups.

As the community engagement guidance is aimed primarily at providers of local services and seeks to address many local issues, it refers to the target group as 'communities' or 'community members'. For the purpose of this chapter this definition has been extrapolated to patient/carer/service user/

community and lay members who would be the 'target population' when implementing the community engagement guidance within NICE. Similarly, this chapter uses the terms 'community engagement' and 'patient involvement' interchangeably to accurately refer to NICE procedures and the guidance itself. NICE involves both individual patients and members of the public and organisations representing their interests. It is acknowledged that there are differences between community engagement and patient involvement in both philosophy and application, but in this context their similarities are more significant than their differences and the terms are intended to be used interchangeably.

NICE COMMUNITY ENGAGEMENT RECOMMENDATIONS

The community engagement guidance puts forward 12 recommendations.[2] These are grouped into four categories, which are intended to be implemented consecutively. *See* box below.

Prerequisites
1 Policy development
2 Long-term investment
3 Organisation and cultural change
4 Levels of engagement and power
5 Mutual trust and respect

Investment
6 Training and resources
7 Partnership working
8 Area-based initiatives

Approaches
9 Community members as agents of change
10 Community workshops
11 Resident consultancy

Evaluation
12 Evaluation

I will now explore each in detail.

COMMUNITY ENGAGEMENT AT NICE

Policy development

NICE has a clear commitment, made explicit in its patient and public involvement policy, to involve patients/carers/service users/community and lay members in its work.[3] All NICE's advisory bodies (standing committees and groups producing clinical and public health guidance) should include at least two lay people in their membership. In addition, patient and community experts and co-optees are invited to give expert evidence or generally contribute to discussions on specific topics at committee meetings. Patients and carers are also involved in other ways such as providing questionnaire responses to inform NICE's Interventional Procedures Advisory Committee (IPAC). *See* Chapter 6 for more information.

NICE also has a single equalities scheme designed to ensure that equalities are considered in all NICE programmes and procedures.[4] This helps NICE to meet its legislative requirements to promote equality and eliminate unlawful discrimination. Part of this scheme includes a commitment to engage with people and organisations with an interest in any of the different strands of equality. This is supported by the work of the NICE equalities forum and is demonstrated through equalities impact assessments.

Long-term investment

NICE has a dedicated Patient and Public Involvement Programme (PPIP) to develop and support opportunities for patient/public involvement across NICE.[5] The team works to recruit patient and lay members to all NICE advisory bodies and provides advice on how NICE teams can work best with patients and lay people, as well as with third-sector organisations. The PPIP also works with the implementation and communications teams at NICE to help ensure that NICE guidance reaches patients and lay people who have an interest in it.

NICE has expertise in community engagement both within PPIP and in other teams. This expertise was strengthened when NICE merged with the Health Development Agency in 2005. As a result, NICE has a good awareness of the nature of community engagement and the appropriate approaches to use.

NICE has also committed resources and implemented a policy to pay an attendance fee to patients, carers and lay people involved in NICE advisory groups and committees. This is in addition to reimbursing the travel and subsistence costs incurred in attending NICE meetings.

Organisation and cultural change, levels of engagement and power and mutual trust and respect

These three recommendations have been assessed jointly as some practice at NICE meets several of the recommendations.

As a public body open to scrutiny and legal challenge, NICE has clear methods and processes that define its work and how that work should be undertaken. These methods and processes are not always the most conducive to facilitating community engagement for reasons such as the short timeframes for consultation or complex processes. However, NICE has taken steps to help organisations and individuals engage with NICE. These steps include:

➤ support and guidance from PPIP

➤ manuals for patient/carer organisations summarising how to get involved in clinical guidelines, technology appraisals and interventional procedures

➤ identifying appropriate levels of engagement for the task at hand, for example

➤ questionnaire-based engagement for the Interventional Procedures Programme; personal testimony from patient experts at Technology Appraisal Committee meetings

➤ developing templates to enable organisations to comment on NICE draft guidance more easily

➤ producing plain English versions of NICE guidance aimed at patients and carers – the *Understanding NICE Guidance* series.

In addition, NICE has a strong commitment to being open and transparent in its work. NICE consults with its stakeholders and the wider public on the methods and processes used to develop its guidance. Although processes vary between programmes at NICE, in general the draft scopes of individual pieces of guidance and the draft guidance itself are subject to public consultation. NICE responds to comments from registered stakeholders and the consultation documents are published on NICE's website. This transparency helps to develop mutual trust and respect between NICE and its stakeholders.

In terms of levels of engagement and power, the community engagement guidance refers to four levels of engagement. NICE covers three of these levels in its work – informing (e.g. dissemination of guidance), consultation (e.g. stakeholders/consultees) and co-production or collaboration (equal membership of advisory groups/committees) – but not delegated power.

The PPIP works closely with the Patients Involved in NICE (PIN) group, which is an independent group made up of members of patient and voluntary organisations who work closely with NICE. The PIN group meets quarterly and has held workshops at the NICE Annual Conference. NICE offers its meeting rooms and facilities to the PIN group and consults with them on changes to processes at NICE. The PIN group also operates a 'buddy scheme' in which individuals and organisations who have worked extensively with NICE assist newly engaged organisations to find the best way for them to input into NICE's work.

Diversity training is a core requirement for all staff at NICE. NICE has developed its own equality scheme and action plan to ensure that equality and diversity issues are considered and embedded in NICE's programmes. In October 2008, NICE held the inaugural meeting of its equality forum to review and develop work in the area of equalities. The forum was attended by representatives of organisations with an interest in equalities, and senior members of NICE staff including two non-executive directors. The views expressed by the forum were compiled into a report that was presented to NICE's Board.

NICE's communication team also commissioned work to review the methods for communicating with and involving seldom-heard groups. This involved using focus groups to elicit the views of several different groups including: older people; people with learning disabilities, mental illness and physical disabilities; Asian men and women; and African and Caribbean men and women.

NICE's communication team has developed an 'I don't speak NICE' campaign to promote the use of clear language and to discourage the use of jargon in NICE documents. This is relevant to many aspects of communication at NICE from email correspondence to published guidance. The campaign is supported by a series of workshops that all NICE staff are encouraged to attend.

Training and resources

NICE has provided resources to support patients, carers and lay members involved in its work. The PPIP runs training days specifically for patient and carer members of clinical guideline development groups and for community members of public health programme development groups. It also provides ongoing support and advice. The Centre for Clinical Practice at NICE runs workshops on health economics – these are open to any members of NICE guideline development groups. Other opportunities for training are provided by NICE as required.

NICE also provides training for NICE staff and external professionals working with lay people on our committees. This training takes the form of presentations for advisory groups/committees, inductions for staff and training sessions for chairs of guideline development groups. To help achieve full organisational and cultural change, NICE plans to further develop training in this area.

Ongoing support for group members is provided by the centre responsible for each work programme and the PPIP. A PPIP lead is assigned to each guidance topic or committee and is responsible for keeping in contact with patients, carers and lay members, providing support and advice as requested, and helping to resolve any issues when they arise.

The PPIP periodically runs workshops for patient/voluntary organisations to inform them about the programmes at NICE and clarify any issues they might have. These sessions also help the PPIP to identify the best strategies for engaging with patient organisations across the different NICE work programmes.

In line with our duties as a public body, under the Disability Discrimination Act NICE aims to meet specific involvement needs. This includes standard physical access, paying the expenses of a carer accompanying a person, providing guidance in different languages and formats on request, and website access for people with visual impairments. In terms of physical provisions, NICE offices are housed in modern office buildings that are accessible by wheelchair. NICE also has an induction loop built into its main meeting rooms and a smaller portable induction loop for smaller meetings to help any attendees with a hearing impairment.

Partnership working

As well as consulting frequently with its stakeholders, NICE is committed to working in partnership with organisations on discrete pieces of work to draw on their expertise in a particular field. For example, NICE has commissioned organisations involved with children and young people to elicit their views to help develop NICE public health guidance. This ensures that the views and preferences of children and young people are fully taken into account in the final recommendations.

Area-based initiatives

Given the national remit of NICE's work it has limited scope to participate in local-level activities. However, the PPIP started working with Local Involvement Networks (LINks) to help NICE engage with local patients and community members who might be interested in NICE's work. NICE's implementation team also works to ensure that guidance is disseminated at a local level through the work of the implementation consultations, LINks and key stakeholder organisations. The PPIP has also attended meetings with local groups, such as cancer networks, to raise awareness of NICE's work at a local level.

Community members as agents of change, community workshops and resident consultancy

These three recommendations are discussed together as some practice at NICE covers several of the recommendations.

In NICE's public health programme, several community members are recruited to each programme development group as full members. In addition, community members are co-opted into programme development group meetings and the meetings of the Public Health Interventions Advisory Committee (PHIAC) to give expert testimony or generally contribute to discussions on the issues around the particular public health intervention being considered.

All NICE's advisory committees have lay member involvement to bring the patient or public perspective to the meetings. Often the appointed lay members will have experience of, or still be involved with, local community groups (e.g.

the local cancer networks, Breathe Easy networks, etc.) and so will be able to bring the local issues to the committees when relevant.

NICE also has a resident group, the Citizens Council, which is intended to represent the demographics of the adult population of England and Wales.[6] The Citizens Council debates issues relevant to NICE's work and provides advice to NICE on social and ethical issues. The results of the Citizens Council's deliberations feed into NICE's *Social Value Judgements* document, which is used by NICE's advisory bodies and working groups to advise on social and ethical considerations when making their decisions.[7]

NICE's Board holds its bi-monthly public board meetings in different parts of the UK to raise awareness of NICE nationally. These meetings are usually well attended by local NHS employees, patients, carers and members of the public who have the opportunity to put questions to the Board.

Evaluation

The PPIP has undertaken a number of small-scale evaluation projects to assess the experiences and outcomes for people involved as lay members on its advisory bodies and working groups. Two recent examples are a survey of patient experts' experiences at technology appraisal committee meetings, and a survey of patient/carer/service users' and chairs' experiences of being involved on clinical guideline development groups. The results of these studies have been presented at key international healthcare conferences such as the 2008 Health Technology Assessment International conference in Vancouver, Canada and the 2008 Guidelines International conference in Helsinki, Finland. As of July 2009, the PPIP team is undertaking an evaluation into the impact of community member engagement on NICE's public health programme development groups.

AREAS FOR DEVELOPMENT
Recognition and feedback

NICE's commitment to openness and transparency means that the public can easily see (via the NICE website) which organisations and lay members have been involved in the production of each piece of guidance. However, feedback from stakeholders, including feedback from participants at the NICE equalities forum, has suggested that NICE needs to do more to demonstrate where the patient and lay input has made a difference to the guidance. Feeding this information back to the public and the organisations and lay members involved will help to counter any accusations of 'tokenism' with regard to patient and lay involvement at NICE. It will also reinforce to the patients, lay people and organisations involved, the value that NICE feels their contributions add to the guidance, and will contribute to better working relationships between NICE and its stakeholders. The PPIP is working with the centres that produce guidance to help them to demonstrate more clearly how the contributions from patients, carers, lay people and organisations have influenced the guidance produced.

Communication

As mentioned earlier in this chapter, NICE has taken a number of steps to improve its communication with patients, carers and the public. However, given the diverse range of work programmes and the differences in methods and processes for each one, engaging with NICE can still be a challenge for external people and organisations. NICE recognises that there is further work to be done and has developed a strategy and committed resources to improve this area of its work. NICE is also committed to adopting a more proactive and interactive communications programme to help people engage with NICE and to disseminate NICE guidance.

Access to information

Access to information can be an issue for patients, carers and lay people sitting on NICE committees and working groups whereas clinicians, public health professionals and academics sitting on the groups often have access to published literature through their institutions. This creates inequalities and power imbalances. Ensuring equity of access to information is a key recommendation in the community engagement guidance. The creation of NHS Evidence, a single web-based portal that provides access to authoritative clinical and non-clinical evidence and best practices, will be a useful tool in helping to address this inequality.[8] NICE will continue to help patients, carers and lay people access the information they need.

CONCLUSION

NICE has made a significant commitment in both financial and policy terms to an inclusive approach in the development of its guidance. With the support of the PPIP, NICE has ensured that there are community engagement/patient involvement opportunities throughout the guidance development process. Resources are committed to supporting both individuals and organisations engaged with NICE, to help develop collaborative and mutually beneficial relationships.

NICE is continually seeking to develop and improve its community engagement work to ensure that the views of patients, carers and community members are central to the guidance it produces. The recommendations made in the community engagement guidance have provided a framework for improvement, which will inform future community engagement activities at NICE.

REFERENCES

1 National Institute for Health and Clinical Excellence. *About Public Health Guidance.* London: NIHCE. Available at: www.nice.org.uk/aboutnice/whatwedo/aboutpublichealthguidance/about_public_health_guidance.jsp (accessed 22 September 2009).

2 National Institute for Health and Clinical Excellence. *Community Engagement, Quick Reference Guide: NICE public health guidance 9.* London: NIHCE; 2008. Available at: www.nice.org.uk/nicemedia/pdf/PH009CommunityEngagementQuickRefGuide.pdf (accessed 22 September 2009).

3 National Institute for Health and Clinical Excellence. *Patient and Public Involvement Policy.* London: NIHCE. Available at: www.nice.org.uk/getinvolved/patientandpublicinvolvement/patientandpublicinvolvementpolicy/patient_and_public_involvement_policy.jsp (accessed 22 September 2009).

4 National Institute for Health and Clinical Excellence. *NICE's Equality Scheme.* London: NIHCE. Available at: www.nice.org.uk/aboutnice/howwework/NICEEqualityScheme.jsp (accessed 22 September 2009).

5 National Institute for Health and Clinical Excellence. *Patient and Public Involvement Programme.* London: NIHCE. Available at: www.nice.org.uk/getinvolved/patientandpublicinvolvement/ppipinvolvementprogramme.jsp (accessed 22 September 2009).

6 National Institute for Health and Clinical Excellence. *Citizens Council Fact Sheet.* London: NIHCE. Available at: www.nice.org.uk/newsroom/factsheets/citizenscouncil.jsp (accessed 22 September 2009).

7 National Institute for Health and Clinical Excellence. *Social Value Judgements: principles for the development of NICE guidance.* 2nd ed. London: NIHCE; 2008. Available at: www.nice.org.uk/media/C18/30/SVJ2PUBLICATION2008.pdf (accessed 22 September 2009).

8 NHS Evidence. *Evidence in Health and Social Care.* London: NIHCE. Available at: www.evidence.nhs.uk (accessed 22 September 2009).

CHAPTER 9

Background to NICE's Citizens Council

Michael Rawlins

I know of no safer repository of the ultimate powers of society than the people themselves. And if we think them not enlightened enough to exercise that control with a wholesome discretion, the remedy is not to take it from them, but to inform their discretion by education.

Thomas Jefferson to William Jarvis (1820)[1]

NICE was established in 1999 to advise, *inter alia*, on the use of new and established interventions in the NHS.[2] In doing so, NICE is required, by its statutory instruments, to take both clinical and cost effectiveness into account.[3,4] Those responsible for formulating NICE's advice therefore have to make judgements about the interpretation of the evidence base (scientific value judgements) as well as what is good for society (social value judgements).[5]

Members of NICE's advisory bodies are appointed, in large part, for their ability to examine the scientific evidence and make scientific judgements. Although the evidence is crucial in informing decisions, it is never enough: scientific judgements are also necessary. Such scientific judgements may consider the validity of particular surrogate markers; or the validity of the findings and if they can be applied to the population as a whole. Members of advisory bodies may have to assess the likely effectiveness of an intervention in particular subgroups even though these may not have been targeted in the relevant clinical trial(s). And they are often required to use their judgement in evaluating the various assumptions that have been used in the economic models of cost effectiveness.

Social values, too, play a critical role if resources are to be distributed fairly. Balancing efficiency and fairness, in a publicly funded healthcare system such as the NHS, requires NICE's decision makers to reflect the views of the public rather than impose their own personal prejudices.[6] The issue for NICE, at the time it was formed, was how these values might be most reliably elicited.

ELICITING THE PUBLIC'S SOCIAL VALUES

Models for eliciting the public's social values are wanting, but various approaches have been advocated.[7] Some claim that this should be the role of either parliament or the current government. Whether parliament has any legitimacy to make social value judgements for the NHS is unclear.[6] Experience suggests that elected politicians find it extraordinarily difficult to do so.

Public meetings are a time-honoured way to sound out public opinion in the NHS. Yet they provide little opportunity for reflection and deliberation; and attendees are often dominated by those with a vested interest in the matter under discussion.

Opinion polls and surveys can elicit the public's immediate preferences on particular issues. However, responses may be coloured by media activity, and there is generally no opportunity for discussion or considered thought. Responses are exquisitely sensitive to the precise manner in which the question is phrased or framed. Polls and surveys do not provide considered views about the complexities of social values.

A better understanding of the reasons behind the public's immediate preferences can be elicited from focus groups, although these are essentially an extension of polling; there are usually only two to four hours available and still not much opportunity for discussion and deliberation.

A more promising approach has been the use of citizens' juries.[7,8] In this technique, between 12 and 15 members of the public are asked a question, often framed as it would be in a criminal trial (i.e. as a charge). The jurors meet over a period of three to four days. They are usually provided with relevant background material and are given the opportunity – as in a criminal trial – to cross-examine expert witnesses. After one or more opportunities to deliberate amongst themselves, they produce a 'verdict'. Coote and Lenaghan showed that British citizens can indeed engage and deliberate on difficult matters related to healthcare; and that they can reach well-argued conclusions.[7]

NICE'S CITIZENS COUNCIL

The critical requirement to elicit the public's social values was appreciated by NICE's Board at the time it was formed. The Board was intrigued by the experience with citizens' juries in the UK but realised that the approach would need to be modified to meet NICE's requirements.

➤ The Board recognised that more participants than are customarily used in citizens' juries would be needed if the Council was to more accurately represent the adult population of England and Wales. The ultimate size (30 members) was a compromise. Any fewer would make it impossible to achieve broad demographic representation. Many more than this would have seriously diminished the prospect of real deliberation between members. The eventual composition of the Council attempted to ensure that its membership reflected, as far as possible, the adult population structure of England and Wales with respect to gender, age, socioeconomic status, ethnicity, disability and geography.

➤ Applications for membership of the Council would be sought from the adult population of England and Wales. Individuals employed in the NHS, private medicine, healthcare industries, or patient advocacy groups would be excluded from joining. The Council would thus reflect the attitudes of the general public rather than those with professional knowledge and experience of healthcare and the NHS.

➤ The Board carefully considered whether to include children and adolescents in the Council. Experience with citizens' juries in the UK suggested that they had not found it easy to contribute in this type of environment.[7] The Board therefore decided, where necessary and appropriate, to explore the views of children and adolescents by other means.

➤ It was decided that the Council should meet twice yearly, for three days at a time, to discuss a particular issue (usually in the form of 'questions') that NICE needed advice on. The format of meetings would include an explanation of the question and the reasons for asking it. Council members would hear evidence from experts with known, and divergent, views on the particular topic. Crucially, sufficient time would be set aside for members to discuss, debate and deliberate. The Council's conclusions would then be presented as a formal report to the Board. The Board emphasised that did not necessarily expect unanimity from the Council in its advice. Rather, it sought the Council to ensure that the reasons of those holding particular views, whether in the minority or the majority, were clearly encapsulated.

➤ The Board agreed that members' travel and accommodation expenses should be met by NICE. Experience with citizens' juries suggested that it was essential to provide members with an attendance allowance in order to encourage applications from self-employed people, or from those with other commitments, such as family, who might otherwise be inhibited from applying.[7] Members would therefore receive a *per diem* of £150 (based on national average daily wage rates).

➤ In order to achieve continuity, the Board decided that rather than assemble a new group for each meeting (the convention for citizens' juries) members would be appointed for three years and one-third would retire each year. This would allow members to gain knowledge of the NHS and the workings of NICE. In addition it would provide sufficient time to gather experience in deliberation, in reaching consensus, and in reviewing reports. By changing the membership each year, it would ensure that one-third of the Council was refreshed with new blood.

➤ The Board was anxious to avoid contaminating members' views with its own prejudices. It was decided, therefore, that NICE's staff would have only limited contact with Council members in order to avoid inadvertently imposing their own views on members ('capture'). The recruitment of members, as well as the organisation and facilitation of meetings, would be contracted to an independent external agency.

➤ Because the Board's approach to deliberative democracy was largely untried, an independent academic organisation was commissioned to evaluate the scheme. This report has subsequently been published – *see* Chapter 14 for more information.[9]

RECRUITMENT

Members were recruited through advertisements in the national and regional media over a four-week period in August and September 2002.[9] Members were recruited and appointed by an independent outside agency. Around 35 000 people expressed an initial interest in being considered for membership, and 4437 returned application forms.

In order to select Council members, population data for England and Wales was used to get the desired demographic profile (*see* Table 9.1) and a shortlist of 350 applicants was created. Individuals from groups least represented in the population were identified. It was felt, in particular, that young or unskilled people might be hardest to recruit. Ten times the number required were chosen at random so, for example, if three young people belonging to a particular group were needed, 30 applications were selected. This process was repeated for each demographic characteristic. An additional 50 applications were selected at random, for the short list, without applying any demographic criteria.

The short-listed applicants were then scrutinised to exclude those who were ineligible and the remainder were contacted by telephone. Some applicants withdrew at this point. The remaining applicants were finally matched, manually, to reflect the demographic characteristics of the English and Welsh populations.

TABLE 9.1: Demographic characteristics of the members of the Citizens Council.

Characteristic	Desired number(s)	Achieved number(s)
Gender:		
Female	15	15
Male	15	15
Age:		
<25 years	3	4
>60 years	6	6
Registered disability	3	3
Ethnic minority	3	4
Geographical distribution:		
North East	1	2
North West	4	4
Yorkshire and Humber	3	2
East	3	3
East Midlands	2	2
West Midlands	3	3
South East	5	4
London	4	3
South West	3	4
Wales	2	3
Occupational status:		
Home, student, unemployed	4	5
Unskilled/partially skilled	6	4
Skilled non-manual	7	8
Skilled manual	8	7
Managerial and technical	4	4
Professional	1	3

REFLECTIONS ON THE COUNCIL AND ITS MEETINGS

Over the decade of its existence, the Council has published 12 reports in response to questions put to it by NICE. These have formed the basis of NICE's document, *Social Value Judgements*, which serves as a guideline for its advisory bodies as they develop NICE guidance.[10]

The Council, itself, still operates as it did at from the start. Three features have been striking. First, people who volunteer for this type of endeavour are unquestionably forthright and unafraid to express their views in a constructive and useful way. Second, at the beginning, some members were clearly suspicious about the motives in establishing the Council. They were pleased to have been invited to take part, but some suspected that they would be used. At best they thought their views would be ignored and at worst they would be expected to endorse decisions that had already been taken. There is no doubt, now, that Council members fully accept that NICE is making a genuine attempt to engage the public through a process of deliberation. Moreover, they appreciate that the results of their deliberations have a significant impact on the NHS. Third, we have all learnt that members of the public, when given the opportunity, can make extraordinary and meaningful contributions. The continuing national and international interest in, and use of, NICE's guidance means that their impact has been greater than any of us imagined at the outset.

REFERENCES

1 Jefferson T. Letter to William Jarvis. 1820. Available at: http://etext.virginia.edu/etcbin/ot2www-jeffquot?specfile=/web/data/jefferson/quotations/www/jeffquot.o2 W&act=surround&offset=107908&tag=6.+The+Safest+Depository&query=william (accessed 22 September 2009).
2 Rawlins MD. In pursuit of quality: the National Institute for Clinical Excellence. *Lancet.* 1999; **353**(9158): 1079–82.
3 *Statutory Instrument 1999 No 220. The National Institute for Clinical Excellence (Establishment and Constitution) Order 1999.* London: Her Majesty's Stationery Office.
4 *Statutory Instrument 1999 No 2219. The National Institute for Clinical Excellence (Establishment and Constitution) Amendment Order 1999.* London: Her Majesty's Stationery Office.
5 Rawlins MD, Culyer AJ. National Institute for Clinical Excellence and its value judgements. *BMJ.* 2004; **329**: 224–7.
6 Rawlins MD. Pharmacopolitics and deliberative democracy. *Clin Med.* 2005; **5**(5): 471–5.
7 Coote A, Lenaghan J. *Citizens' Juries: theory into practice.* London: Institute for Public Policy Research; 1997.
8 Stewart J, Kendall E, Coote A. *Citizens's Juries.* London: Institute for Public Policy Research; 1994.
9 Davies C, Wetherell M, Barnett E, *et al. Opening the Box: evaluating the Citizens Council of NICE. Report prepared for the National Coordinating Centre for Research Methodology, NHS Research and Development Programme.* Milton Keynes: The Open University; March 2005.
10 National Institute for Health and Clinical Excellence. *Social Value Judgements: principles for the development of NICE guidance.* 2nd ed. London: NIHCE; 2008.

CHAPTER 10

Ordinary people, extraordinary wisdom

Ela Pathak-Sen

In this chapter, I will describe how we, the facilitators, worked with the Citizens Council to answer questions posed by NICE. I will describe our interventions and methodology but more importantly seek to share our learning along the way. We had two important aspects to our work: keeping the Citizens Council members engaged; and facilitating a useful response to NICE's questions.

RECRUITING AND KEEPING MEMBERS ENGAGED

Our first job was recruiting the 'right' 30 people to the Council and helping them realise that they had something important to contribute. The first advertisement we ran had a bold caption: 'Have your say in the NHS'. The response was overwhelming, far greater than we expected. At a time when it was thought the public was disengaged from politics and social issues, we learnt that this was not the case. The public seemed to have quite a lot to say about the NHS and saw this as their opportunity to fix their local hospital or GP surgery. Our telephone lines were jammed and our postbox full. We had 35 000 requests for information and these converted into over 4000 applications. The NICE brief was very clear: 30 ordinary members of the public from all walks of life but with no links to the NHS. We were set the task of finding a disinterested but interested public.

Applying had to be easy, especially if we wanted to encourage those who would not normally pursue a formal application. We kept the application form simple and allowed people to tell us about how they had dealt with challenging issues. We heard a plethora of stories about individuals pursuing their dreams, fighting for big and little causes, or just getting by. We developed a demographic profile in conjunction with NICE to try and gain a cross-section of the population. We used computerised random and focused selection methods. Our final 30 successful applicants included a London taxi driver, a single mum from Tyne and Wear, a retired airline pilot and a local government officer from Middlesex.

The plan was for members to come together for two meetings a year. We started by holding meetings around the country. Our first meeting was in Salford, followed by Cardiff, Sheffield and then Brighton. The idea was that we would take the meetings to the people, hold them in public, and as far as possible, use public spaces to do this. In Cardiff and Hove we met in the Council Chambers, for example. Our main challenge was getting the members to these meetings. We made all travel arrangements for Council members – our perspective being that the less stressful we made this for individuals, the more likely they would attend. We had to take account of access issues, and not just for those who required special arrangements because of certain disabilities; we also needed to consider members who had never travelled as far as we expected them to, and for whom funding a train ticket (even though they would be reimbursed) made a difference as to whether or not they could attend.

We started with a two-day induction in London and the Council members met the Board of NICE and began to find out more about NICE's work – up till then, for a number of members, viewpoints about NICE had been shaped purely by the popular press. There were three elements to the initial induction, the first was to test out whether or not the newly recruited members felt able to contribute and continue, the second was to help them understand NICE's work, and the third was to make members aware that this was an experiment and that it was likely to attract media attention. For us as facilitators, it was the first opportunity to gauge the various interaction styles of the individuals and their preferred learning style, and to plan our strategy to get them through the stages of group formation.[1] We also learnt to be prepared to review our group-building techniques following the introduction of 10 new members whenever the Council was refreshed.

What became apparent at this initial induction was that our role as Council's friend was very important. We had already spent considerable time on the phone to individual members before the meeting reassuring, advising and helping sort travel and childcare arrangements – our primary focus being on getting them to come to the induction. Once at induction we had to reassure the different factions that quickly emerged. There were those who had never experienced what they considered a formal meeting structure and therefore did not know the rules, and there were others who thought they understood the rules and were slightly disconcerted when they discovered that 'normal' rules did not apply. We were very keen for the members to understand and be assured that all experience counted; we did not want their views hampered by 'committee-speak' or political correctness.

We used the usual facilitative techniques of getting the group to set ground rules, but we also explored with them what this might mean. As facilitators we had to be prepared to accept that on occasion opinions would stray into uncomfortable, edgy areas and we had to be ready to manage this. For example, on the last day of our first meeting one of the younger members of the group said she felt frustrated because she felt that minority groups had their rights protected whilst, because she was perceived to belong to the majority, she felt penalised. Our role as facilitators was not to close this conversation down but to try to help her express it in a way that allowed members of minority groups the opportunity to listen and to express how it felt from their perspective. This led to a facilitated session at the start of the next meeting on managing the whole area of equality. We wanted members to say how they felt, but in a way that didn't attack other members of the group. This wasn't easy; we experienced the whole gamut of feelings from not wanting to be preached at, to not wanting to be made an example of. We carried on because we felt this had to be done. Interestingly, after that session the group began to 'police' themselves whilst we kept a watchful eye!

WHAT DID NICE WANT THE CITIZENS COUNCIL TO DO?

NICE explained to the Citizens Council (and those watching the experiment) that it had set up the Council to help it deliberate on social value judgements. NICE described how its work required it to make judgements on clinical and cost effectiveness. It was our job as facilitators to translate this to the Citizens Council while NICE had the job of translating it to the wider world.

It was interesting grappling with the language during those first months. As one Citizens Council member put it: 'What's a social value judgement when it's at home?' And another member said after the induction: 'But what are we going to actually do; how will our decision affect the NHS?' Almost all public debate in health up to that time had focused on specific issues: what treatments should we provide; what should we pay for; should a hospital close and the like. We were truly in uncharted territory; on the one hand the public view of NICE was about saying yes or no to drugs and on the other, NICE was asking the Council to contribute to the debate that underpinned what NICE should say yes and no to, and why. NICE explained this by saying that it gathered the clinical, economic and patient experts to contribute to the decision making based on their expertise. NICE recognised that value judgements required a different kind of expertise, and who better than a group of 'ordinary people drawn from all walks of life'.

SETTING THE QUESTIONS

NICE established a subcommittee of the Board to oversee the Citizens Council and to develop the questions. The first question was the hardest to set and there was much discussion on whether it was better to start with a general question and move to more-focused ones, or to move from the particular to the general. NICE decided that the former was more appropriate, hence the first question on clinical need: 'What should NICE take into account when making decisions about clinical need?'

In hindsight, perhaps NICE was being too optimistic in expecting a full answer to this question. When Sir Michael Rawlins opened the first meeting with the remark that experts had found it difficult to define clinical need, the new Council members – far from rising to the challenge – were perplexed. If experts and learned people in their field had not yet answered the question, what hope was there for 30 members of the public to do so in three days? And then the doubts crept in: the Council was not answering questions directly about services in the NHS; how exactly would their work contribute to the NHS; was this some ploy to make NICE look good?

As facilitators, we had to let this run its course. Any attempt to speak for NICE would mean that in the eyes of the Council we were biased. At early meetings NICE kept its distance. Sir Michael Rawlins opened the meetings and the project manager observed them, but other than those who presented information on behalf of NICE, the Council was left to deliberate the question with the expert speakers and the facilitators. This had its advantages because it demonstrated NICE's sincerity in truly seeking a view unsullied by NICE. However, the disadvantage was that when there was uncertainty around the question, or facts about NICE, this was difficult to clarify. It was later decided to hold the meetings at NICE's offices in London but with the facilitators maintaining distance between NICE and the Council. This allowed NICE staff to be available to clarify unclear questions or provide factual background.

Setting the subsequent questions got easier. NICE had a better sense of what it wanted to ask and how it was going to use the answers it heard, and we understood how the individuals worked and were able to frame the questions in language the Council members understood. We adopted a number of helpful techniques. For example, we would test questions with a random sample of the public to check if they were understandable. We also agreed that the Council members would have the opportunity to comment on the draft question. This had the added advantage of gaining their buy-in to the meeting, and members could check ambiguity before the meeting and also recommend speakers to the facilitators.

DRAWING UP THE AGENDA

The facilitators worked with NICE to draw up the agenda for the meetings. The basic outline was adapted from the citizens' jury model.[2,3] Time was allocated for explaining the question, providing arguments for and against possible answers, cross-questioning, and for debate and discussion. As the format developed over time, we learnt that we needed to provide enough structure to eliminate uncertainty whilst maintaining enough flexibility to allow members to explore the areas and issues they wanted to. The temptation was to overload the programme with expert speakers, because we wanted the members to have enough information and opinions to be able to explore the various angles of the argument during their discussions. The problem with this was, of course, time – sufficient time for the speakers so that they felt their view had been heard; time for the members to absorb the ideas and cross-question the speakers; and time to deliberate. The other problem was ensuring we had speakers who could represent both sides of the argument. More often than not, it was easier to find those who agreed with the topic or question than those who were against it. Initially we did worry about whether or not we had got the balance right, but as the process matured both facilitators and NICE became more relaxed about this. And we learnt to trust the Citizens Council.

It became very important to prepare the experts for the meetings. Most experts in their field are of course used to public speaking and presenting but to a very different audience, compared with the Citizens Council. Before every meeting we spent time briefing the speakers, talking through the programme, putting ourselves in the members' shoes, ensuring that they would be understood by all the members, but mostly reassuring them. It was uplifting to watch world experts trying to succinctly explain some very complex concepts to this diverse cross-section of the general public while they pushed back, testing, honing and refining their positions, unafraid to challenge. This does not mean that everything was understood all of the time. Some concepts just had to be worked at. The question of quality-adjusted life years is a moot point for example. This came to the fore at the second and third meetings when the issue of age was tackled[4] and was a recurring theme throughout the meetings. We knew the concept was going to be hard to get across so we constructed a few case studies where the members did a role-play exercise to represent the NICE decision-making groups. As we tackled different topics through the meetings we realised a couple of things. The first was that the members themselves built up a store of accumulated knowledge that they tested out in their daily lives between meetings and they passed this knowledge on to new members. Second, we learnt that as facilitators we should review certain concepts to give members a deeper understanding to apply to their deliberations. We had to vary the way in which we did this: providing information sheets for new members at induction, briefing notes before meetings, and mini tutorials from NICE staff. But by far and away the best method was experiential learning and we had to make space on the programme for this to happen.

We also needed to make space for quiet reflection and small-group deliberation. There was a danger that we would overload the programme with expert speakers and case studies and that the morning of the third day would result in hurried discussion. To enable us to keep track of the members thinking we introduced tracking questionnaires to take soundings at the beginning and end of each day. We could then adapt our approach and the programme if we saw patterns emerging. We also summarised the discussions at the beginning and end of the day in a report. For the first few meetings the lead facilitator wrote the report on behalf of the Citizens Council. We later agreed with NICE to use an expert reporter to record the meetings so that the lead facilitator could concentrate on facilitating.

RUNNING THE MEETING

Each meeting began with a welcome from Sir Michael Rawlins and Professor Peter Littlejohns, followed by an explanation of how NICE had taken into account the recommendations from the previous report. Two Citizens Council members always had an opportunity to present the report at a Board meeting and the rest of the Council were eager to check process. The Citizens Council maintained an element of healthy cynicism and a need to know that what they were doing was useful. As once Council member put it: 'How many nurses would our meetings fund? – I really want to know if what we are doing is worthwhile'.

For the first few meetings this was hard to explain as NICE was still considering the best way to make use of the reports from the Citizens Council. However, NICE was open about this and so the members persevered. In 2005, Sir Michael Rawlins published the first edition of NICE's *Social Value Judgements* paper and the members had a clearer idea on what was going to happen with their work.[5] However, it wasn't until the second edition that NICE formalised the process of asking its decision-making committees to demonstrate that they had taken into account the social value judgements endorsed by the Board.[6] That some of the Citizens Council members continued to contribute despite their uncertainty, is a testament to NICE's openness and transparency with them.

The first part of each meeting was spent introducing the question. Citizens Council members had the opportunity to test their understanding of the question with NICE and this was followed by presentations to help set the context. Facilitators were on hand to help members 'frame' questions if this was required. A useful approach to managing multiple presenters was to set up a 'question time' panel based on the popular BBC Question Time programme. Presenters were given a maximum of 10 minutes to state their case and the lead facilitator moderated questions from the members as well as questions between the panel. This generated a lively debate between the panel members and was very productive.

One of the challenges of facilitating a large group is to try and make sure that 'quieter' voices are heard. Throughout the day we tracked those who had spoken and those who hadn't and checked with the quieter ones if they felt they were able to speak up. We recognised that for some members speaking in smaller groups was more comfortable, whereas others required help to frame their questions and wanted to use facilitators as a sounding board to clarify their thoughts. We had to tread carefully between working to empower members to speak for themselves, and negotiating and speaking for them when necessary.

In our early meetings we realised that the agenda balance between expert opinion and members' opinions was unequal, with more time being given to expert opinion. It was also apparent that relying on expert opinion pushed the members' thinking down a particular route. This resulted in rushed and sometimes highly-charged opinions on the final day with limited opportunity to test these out. To counteract this, we began using open space technology on the second and third day.[7] This had the effect of getting the members to flag and focus on issues that were important to them and also allowed them to take charge of the discussion. It meant that on the last day we focused on highlighting areas of agreement and disagreement. We made it clear to members that we were not looking for consensus; we were interested in hearing majority and minority views, but more importantly we needed to understand why these views were held. We wanted to make absolutely sure that members left the meeting having clearly stated what their key response to NICE was.

The report was written in the two weeks following the meeting and comments were invited from the members via email. If email was difficult or unavailable to members, we sent out hard copies and telephoned them to record their comments. Only when the Citizens Council had agreed the content of the report was it presented to NICE. On occasion NICE sought clarification and this was provided before the report was published.

WHAT DID WE LEARN?

Some of what we learnt about facilitating was not new, rather it reinforced our thinking about people's behaviour be they a diverse group of the public or an expert panel well versed in the art of deliberation. We learnt about risk taking and experimenting in a very public arena and how experiments like this are only possible with commitment and support from the very top of the commissioning organisation. The question we have asked ourselves is 'What would we do differently?' A key area for us would be to create greater certainty about what NICE was going to ask the Citizens Council and how the information was going to be used. But this was an experiment and NICE too was treading fairly uncharted waters. The Citizens Council members felt supported by the NICE Board and in particular Sir Michael Rawlins.

Setting up an iterative evaluation at the start of the process was incredibly helpful for us as facilitators and assisted our learning at every meeting.[8]

Most importantly we learnt about trust and 'ordinary' people. We were reminded that there are no such things as 'ordinary' people, just extraordinary people doing ordinary things. Creating the right environment and creating an atmosphere of trust means that a group of citizens can consider and deliberate complex issues and contribute to public decision making.

REFERENCES

1 Tuckman BW, Jensen MAC. Stages of small-group development revisited. *Group & Organisation Management.* 1977; 2(4): 419–27.

2 Coote A, Lenaghan J. *Citizens' Juries: theory into practice.* London: Institute for Public Policy Research; 1997.

3 Davies S, Elizabeth S, Hanley B. *Ordinary Wisdom: reflections on an experiment in citizenship and health.* London: Kings Fund; 1998.

4 National Institute for Health and Clinical Excellence. *NICE Citizens Council Report on Age.* London: NIHCE; 2005. Available at: www.nice.org.uk/nicemedia/pdf/Citizenscouncil_report_age.pdf (accessed 22 September 2009).

5 National Institute for Health and Clinical Excellence. *Social Value Judgements: principles for the development of NICE guidance.* London: NIHCE; 2005. Available at: www.nice.org.uk/media/873/2F/SocialValueJudgementsDec05.pdf (accessed 22 September 2009).

6 National Institute for Health and Clinical Excellence. *Social Value Judgements: principles for the development of NICE guidance.* 2nd ed. London: NIHCE; 2008. Available at: www.nice.org.uk/media/C18/30/SVJ2PUBLICATION2008.pdf (accessed 22 September 2009).

7 Harrison O. *Open Space Technology: a user's guide.* San Francisco: Berrett-Koehler; 1992.

8 Davies C, Wetherell M, Barnett E, et al. *Opening the Box: evaluating the Citizens Council of NICE. Report prepared for the National Coordinating Centre for Research Methodology, NHS Research and Development Programme.* Milton Keynes: The Open University; March 2005.

CHAPTER 11

The Citizens Council reports

Peter Littlejohns

The inaugural Citizens Council meeting took place in Salford in November 2002 and the latest meeting was held in June 2009 in London. There have been 12 meetings during this period that have covered the topics:

➤ clinical need
➤ age
➤ confidential enquiries
➤ ultra-orphan drugs
➤ mandatory public health measures
➤ rule of rescue
➤ health inequalities
➤ only in research
➤ patient safety
➤ quality-adjusted life years (QALYs) and the severity of illness
➤ departing from the threshold
➤ the nature of innovation.

The full reports (including the questions posed, the agendas, speakers and accompanying documents) are available on the NICE website.[1]

In this chapter, I will provide an overview of the type of questions NICE has asked the Citizens Council to address, and a summary of its responses.

In many ways the type of questions NICE has asked reflects its development over the first 10 years since its inception and the challenges it has faced. The questions are a mixture of very-broad-brush questions on the nature of healthcare itself, such as the first question posed to the Council on 'determining clinical need', and more specific questions, such as the ethical basis of analysing patient data when the patient has not given consent.

PREPARING THE QUESTIONS

Prior to the first Citizens Council meeting, NICE's internal and external stake-holders convened in a dedicated workshop to determine the questions. The questions are now determined by the Citizens Council Committee, which is a subcommittee of the NICE Board. The Committee meets periodically to iden-tify the issues facing NICE and its advisory bodies in making decisions. It then formulates the exact question that needs to be asked. Over the years the way of presenting the question has continued to evolve but it usually consists of setting the question in a social and ethical setting.

Once the question has been determined, the Committee, in conjunction with external facilitators, prepares the agenda for the three days. External speak-ers, usually from both sides of the argument, are invited to outline the issues to the Council and time is allocated to small-group work and deliberation.

In the early days the facilitators prepared summary reports of the Council meetings. However, more recently a medical journalist, Geoff Watts, has attended the meetings and captured the deliberations as they have proceeded. He then prepares a report, which gets approved by the Council before being presented to the public NICE Board Meeting by two Citizens Council members.

FIRST REPORT OF THE CITIZENS COUNCIL: CLINICAL NEED

In some ways the first meeting report was unique as it responded to a very gen-eral question, but one that is fundamental to NICE's work in assessing clinical effectiveness. When presented with the issue of 'clinical need', the Citizens Council soon identified the necessity to expand the 'narrow' concept of the 'need for medical intervention' to include the social environment in which care is provided.

They were clear on the features of the disease that should be taken into account:

'In the Council's opinion the following (in no specific order) are the most important features of a disease, or condition, that should be taken into account when deciding clinical need:

➤ How bad is the pain and how severe are the symptoms?
➤ Is it potentially fatal?
➤ Is it contagious?
➤ Are there no alternative treatments available?
➤ What is the long-term effect of the condition on the individual?
➤ What are the chances of a good clinical outcome?
➤ What is the number of patients affected?
➤ What is the effect of the disease on the quality of life for the individual patient?
➤ What is the effect of the disease on the length of life for the individual?

- What are the psychological effects of the condition?
- What is the level of disability and/or independence of the individual?
- Is the condition time limited?
- Are there fluctuations in the individual's condition?
- Is the disease or the condition cosmetic?
- What are the side effects encountered by the patient?
- Is there any stigma related to the condition?
- What are the resources available, such as cost and equipment?'

But the Council also concluded that the characteristics of the patient are important:

'In the Council's opinion the following (in no specific order) are the most important features of patients, rather than their condition, that should be taken into account when deciding clinical need:
- What values does the patient have?
- What is the patient's ability to make an informed decision?
- What is the age of the patient?
- How fit is the patient to undergo treatment?
- What are the patient's other conditions?
- How able is the patient to self-manage their condition?
- What is the family history, and are there any genetic or hereditary issues for the patient?
- Has a holistic approach for the patient been considered?'

The Council was clear that some features should *not* be considered in determining need including:
- social and economic factors
- whether it is a 'self-induced' disease or condition
- how loud the 'voice' of the patient is
- a patient's ethnic background, sex or location.

The most important directive to NICE was that when a patient had in any way contributed to their illness, this should not be a consideration in deciding on treatment, although the Councillors still suggested that if ongoing behaviour seriously influenced the effectiveness of an intervention then its continued use should be reconsidered.

SECOND REPORT OF THE CITIZENS COUNCIL: AGE

When considering the first question on clinical need the Citizens Council identi-fied that individuals at different ages require different levels of care and this was reflected in their response. However, because of how this view was presented in the first report, some commentators interpreted it as being 'ageist'. NICE therefore invited the Citizens Council to explore the issue of 'age' in healthcare more closely at its next meeting.

The majority of the Council concluded that when NICE is deciding what constitutes 'value for money' to the NHS and when age is an indicator of risk, it is legitimate – indeed vital in some circumstances – to differentiate by age. However, the Council did not think that NICE should be more generous to some age groups than others on the basis of social roles that people have at different ages.

Perhaps most importantly they were exposed to the 'fair innings' argument by its originator, the late Professor Alan Williams. He presented his thesis that 'older people' who had had a long life should be prepared to take a smaller proportion of healthcare resources than the young who were just starting their life – less money for the grandparent to allow more for the grandchild. As eloquent as Alan was, the Citizens Council was not persuaded by his argument. Most members did not think that the NHS should be more generous in its definition of what constitutes value for money for certain age groups based on people's life experience opportunities due to their age.

Age is one of the key items in NICE's social value principles and it counsels advisory committees to value one year of life equally at all ages. However in January 2009, NICE issued further recommendations to its advisory committees stating that in some circumstances, for small patient groups when life expectancy is known to be very short and new treatments represent a 'step change' compared to existing treatment, a more generous interpretation of 'value for money' should be applied.

THIRD REPORT OF THE CITIZENS COUNCIL: CONFIDENTIAL ENQUIRIES

At the time of this meeting, NICE was responsible for the National Confidential Enquiries ('Enquiries'). These are long-standing professional groupings that assess patient deaths and seek to learn lessons that can feed back into the healthcare system to improve the quality of patient care. At the time of the meeting, their continued existence was under threat due to new legislation that would require them to seek patient consent. As the patients whose care was being assessed were already dead, consent could be obtained only from the next of kin and obtaining this quickly without causing further anguish to the relatives would be difficult. Temporary exemption was in place but would not last forever.

NICE wanted to know what the public's attitude was to the Enquiries use of patient information obtained from medical records, and asked the Citizens Council to discuss this issue.

The key findings were that the Citizens Council thought that the Enquiries make an important contribution to healthcare. Most members did not think the Enquiries should be required to seek individual informed consent before using medical records for their research. More than two-thirds of the Council felt strongly that the arguments for gaining consent were offset by the benefits to the public of the work of the Enquiries. Most accepted that it would be impractical to require it to seek such consent: they felt it could compromise the quality of the research, place an unsustainable burden on the Enquiries, and divert resources from other parts of the NHS. Most accepted that it is currently impractical to require hospitals to make all data completely anonymous at source, and overall most of them were satisfied as to the security and confidentiality of the pseudo-anonymous data used by the Enquiries.

Generally speaking, their objections were on the grounds of impracticality, not intrusiveness to the individuals concerned. They acknowledged that although such conversations would not be easy, medical professionals deal with sensitive situations all the time, and most people accept that in the event of the death of a loved one, some things are essential even if they are distressing.

However, a minority believed that it is essential that the Enquiries *should* seek consent, on the grounds that it is not right to make use of information about individuals without their express permission. Even if there is a good case for the NHS needing that information in the interests of the greater good, some members of the Council felt strongly that it is not acceptable to assume that it can be used without reference to the patient or their next of kin.

On balance, the Citizens Council supported the case put by the Enquiries that they should not be required to seek individual informed consent. They also felt that there were a number of important culture changes that needed to take place – both within the Enquiries and the NHS as a whole.

First, it was noted that prior to the meeting only one member of the Citizens Council was aware of the existence of the Enquiries. This was a matter of concern, and the Council wanted to see NICE, the Enquiries and the NHS do much more to make the public aware of the organisation, its use of patient records, and the impact of their results on the development of healthcare in the NHS.

The Council felt that once the public knew about the work of the Enquiries, they would be more likely – not less – to support the use of their records for developing better practice, and for learning from and addressing system failure. Although the Council recognised that the Enquiries undertook good work, it was not acceptable that the public didn't know it was happening. Regardless of where any of the Council members stood on the need to gain informed consent for the use of medical records, they all felt it was vital that the public was more aware that these processes take place.

Some of the Citizens Council thought that it would be possible to avoid the need to seek individual informed consent by undertaking a widespread publicity campaign. This would ensure that the public was made aware of the work of the Enquiries, and of the use that some patients' medical records might be put to in the pursuit of this work. In this way, it was suggested that general consent could be assumed to have been given, unless an individual chose to 'opt out' and have their medical records marked as such. The Council thought the introduction of the electronic patient record might make this easier in practice, but some members felt it might be possible already.

All members of the Citizens Council supported the concept of a learning NHS. However, they believed that in order for everyone to benefit from ever-improving healthcare, there needed to be systems in place to encourage honest disclosure of events. The Council believed this was not just a matter for health professionals and that the systems should be continually reviewed with the aim of doing more to encourage patients and the public to get involved in helping improve the NHS. It suggested that this may be part of a culture change from paternalism to partnership.

Citizens Council discussions often refer to the responsibilities as well as the rights that patients, the public as a whole and health professionals have.

Much was made of the reciprocal arrangements assumed between individuals and a national health service. As one Council member said: 'We take a great deal from the NHS – why not say thank you by putting something back?'

But there was debate between members as to what this implied, and whether it should be made more explicit as part of the patients' charter. The Council believed that people need to know more about how the NHS works, and what their role is in relation to it. Regardless of Council members' personal views on whether individual consent was required in this instance, the entire Council wanted the NHS to adopt a greater culture of openness and to trust the public.

The second desired cultural change related to the fact that members were not aware of the history and the context in which relationships between the public and the medical profession had developed over the years. Some of the members of the Citizens Council were not entirely convinced that when they are told something is 'impossible' or 'impracticable', it isn't actually because the professionals think it is 'difficult' or 'inconvenient' for them. Many wanted to see a more 'can do' attitude in relation to finding ways to involve the public in making decisions about how their data is used and about healthcare right across the board. It was not so long ago that patients were told it was impossible to see their own medical records.

Most members of the Citizens Council felt that they would like the opportunity for them, as a Citizens Council (or for the public as a whole), to review the situation in the future once the use of new technology, such as electronic patient records, opened up new possibilities for the storage and sharing of information. They suspected their views could change in the future, if new technology made alternative arrangements possible. However, a review should not necessarily be limited to a time when there is an integrated electronic system within the NHS.

The Council was also convinced that informed debate amongst the public can only strengthen the support that individuals give to the system of collective provision that is the NHS. Some members felt very strongly that we couldn't expect, as individuals, to opt out of one part of a system and then expect the system as a whole to be there for us when we need it.

Even those who supported the idea of people being able to 'opt out' on an individual basis hoped that this option would be exercised in only a tiny proportion of cases. While a minority of the Council thought that the individual right to withhold consent is an important principle to safeguard for others, none said they were likely to exercise it for themselves.

Finally, a number of members noted that the NHS has changed substantially since the Enquiries started and there are now other organisations – not least the National Patient Safety Agency – that have been set up to help the NHS learn and improve. While the Council supported this work, some members suggested that it's possible that some of the difficulties involved in 'sharing' data might be avoided if the NHS acted as more of a coherent whole.

FOURTH REPORT OF THE CITIZENS COUNCIL: ULTRA-ORPHAN DRUGS

The Citizens Council was asked to advise on whether the NHS should be prepared to pay premium prices for drugs to treat patients with very rare diseases. Twenty-seven members of the Citizens Council met to discuss this in November 2004.

The report from the meeting concluded:

'Everyone approached this discussion from the point of view of wanting to do what's fair – but we have different ideas on fairness. Twenty of us have taken a decision that we should use a different way of assessing value – 16 give a qualified 'yes' when it comes to paying for ultra-orphan drugs, and four think that there shouldn't be conditions attached. Seven of us feel that rare diseases should not have a different decision-making process applied to them.'

The main criteria that the Citizens Council thought the NHS should take into account when deciding to pay premium prices for ultra-orphan drugs were, in descending order of importance:

➤ the degree of severity of the disease
➤ whether the disease or condition is life threatening
➤ whether the treatment will provide health gain, rather than just stabilisation of the condition.

NICE's current position on this issue, in accordance with Department of Health advice, is to apply its normal processes to drugs that the Department of Health refers, whatever the size of the patient population. However, the Department of Health will normally avoid referring drugs used only for very small patient groups.

FIFTH REPORT OF CITIZENS COUNCIL: MANDATORY PUBLIC HEALTH MEASURES

In 2005, NICE took on the functions of the Health Development Agency and therefore the responsibility to provide guidance on disease prevention and health promotion as well as disease management. This can involve applying a different set of values so the Citizens Council was asked to consider when they thought it appropriate that mandatory rather than voluntary approaches to public health should be invoked.

In their deliberations, the Citizens Council formed principles to deal with a number of issues as outlined below (with the accompanying points to consider and other perspectives).

WHO HAS RESPONSIBILITY FOR THE PUBLIC'S HEALTH – INDIVIDUALS OR THE STATE?

Principles

The Council concluded that, where possible, people should have freedom of choice and be responsible for their own health. The state should attempt to educate people to adopt a healthier lifestyle and try to persuade them to voluntarily access the help they need. But ultimately, and if necessary, it should adopt mandatory measures.

Freedom of choice is overridden by the responsibility to not cause harm to others. Where others are being harmed by a particular activity the state has a right to intervene.

Points to consider

An individual whose behaviour deliberately puts others at risk could face legal penalties.

Other perspectives

Six Council members thought that public health interventions should target problems that affect the majority, as well as problems affecting minorities.

WHERE DOES THE BALANCE LIE BETWEEN NEEDS AND BENEFITS VERSUS HARM AND INCONVENIENCE?

Principles

The Council concluded that any mandatory measure should lead to overall improvement in the health of the population.

Interventions that provide benefit for the greater number are justified even where a small minority might be disadvantaged.

Minor inconvenience resulting from an intervention should have little bearing on whether or not it is made mandatory.

Finally, mandatory measures should lead to worthwhile benefits compared to the cost. A broad view needs to be taken of costs and benefits as some may not be immediately apparent.

Points to consider

Care should be taken that interventions address a genuine public health problem rather than the latest media fad.

Other perspectives

Most of the Council supported interventions that offer benefit to significant numbers of the population 'even when a small minority might be disadvantaged'. However, two members disagreed. One member was concerned about the disproportionate impact that even worthwhile interventions might have on businesses and small enterprises.

The majority of the Council emphasised that preventive health must be adopted on its own merits and should not be seen as a way of avoiding proper spending on acute services.

One Council member felt that the degree of disadvantage considered acceptable, when introducing an intervention, might need to be defined further. 'If the intervention could cause the death of some people, is it still OK?'

WHEN AND HOW SHOULD THE STATE INTERVENE?

Principles

The Council thought the choice of intervention should be based on the seriousness of the problem, the extent of harm or danger within the population and the number of people it would affect.

The Council accepted that the quality of the evidence needed to justify a public health intervention might be lower in the case of an urgent national emergency, for example bird flu or bio-terrorism.

There was consensus that mandatory public health measures should aim to promote equality of outcome. The Council acknowledged that this may mean treating some people differently from others in order to reduce health inequalities.

The Council noted that potential adverse effects of a mandatory public health intervention on vulnerable members of society should always be considered.

Points to consider

If the condition being addressed is common, the Council thought it is right to target the intervention at the most vulnerable groups. For example, flu vaccinations are targeted at older people and those most likely to suffer serious side effects if they get flu.

Interventions should attempt to address the *cause* of a public health problem (e.g. promoting healthy foods to children) as well as focusing on the *symptoms* of the problem (e.g. prescribing exercise for already obese people).

Other perspectives

Whilst many of the Council members were concerned that measures should address the cause of the problem as well as the symptom, others pointed out that this might not always be possible either because of the problem's complexity (e.g. obesity) or its urgency (e.g. treating an outbreak of bird flu). The Council agreed that these difficulties should not put a promising intervention at risk: 'Sometimes the cause may be very hard to address, such as psychological origins of overeating, and the best you can do is treat the symptom.'

A majority of members felt it was important to openly acknowledge if someone suffered an adverse effect and to provide compensation. But four members disagreed and believed this only encouraged the 'compensation culture'.

More than half of the Council felt exemptions should be allowed for certain groups on the grounds of, for instance, religious belief, so long as it did not influence the effectiveness of the intervention as a whole. But a minority disagreed, feeling this would inevitably dilute its effectiveness. 'Too many opt outs can cause apathy amongst those who cannot opt out,' was one comment.

But some members disagreed and others were undecided. One person pointed out that dental fluorosis, the one agreed side effect of fluoridation, did not amount to harm or danger but should still be taken into account.

Three members opposed giving preferential treatment to the most vulnerable, largely on the grounds of impracticality. One felt that mandatory measures should apply to all equally. There were also doubts about treating some people differently to others in order to narrow the inequalities gap.

Others questioned the practicality of treating everyone impartially. 'While you should not gratuitously discriminate against any person or groups, in some public health issues you need to treat people differently in order to help them.'

HOW SHOULD MANDATORY INTERVENTIONS BE INTRODUCED AND MONITORED?

Principles

The Council concluded that any mandatory measure should be monitored, once implemented. If monitoring reveals significant harmful consequences, the measure should be reconsidered in order to limit damage.

Where vulnerable groups are at risk, monitoring should be particularly rigorous.

Points to consider

It was noted that mandatory measures should be introduced only if they are practical and achievable.

Wherever possible, the Citizens Council thought measures should be piloted first before being extended to the whole country.

It also believed there should be a provision to review and stop the measure in the future if it turned out to be unfavourable. It was important to the Council that measures were reversible.

Other perspectives

Two members were doubtful about making practicality one of the tests of whether to introduce a measure: 'if it is serious enough to warrant mandatory measures it must be made to work' was one comment; 'sometimes we will only know this after a period of time has elapsed' was another.

Whilst the Citizens Council members generally supported piloting interventions, a few of them were concerned that pilots would involve some people being treated like 'guinea pigs'. In some cases there might not be time to run a pilot. All agreed on the desirability of research in advance, but essential interventions should not be delayed because of a lack of detailed evidence. This made some members anxious that the effect of an intervention might be undermined if some groups were allowed to opt out.

OPENNESS, TRUST AND PUBLIC INVOLVEMENT

Principles

The Council thought there must be openness and transparency in implementing mandatory measures and in explaining the reasons behind them.

Wherever possible, public health interventions should be preceded by public information and/or consultation, debate and feedback.

Other perspectives

Most of the Council members also felt it was important to consider whether a measure had enough support to make its imposition practical. But six members disagreed. Several pointed out that many successful public health measures, such as compulsory seatbelts and the breathalyser, were extremely unpopular when first introduced.

Several members were unhappy about linking implementation to prior public support, pointing out that sometimes a measure can be both unpopular and right – there are a number of instances where people accept a measure after its implementation even though they didn't before (e.g. drink-driving laws).

One member was opposed to automatic public consultation, noting that often it served only to inflame the situation: 'It may be unhelpful, costly and simply act to heighten fears over what is really common sense.'

SIXTH CITIZENS COUNCIL REPORT: RULE OF RESCUE

NICE's questions on this occasion were:

'Is there a preference to save the life of people in imminent danger of dying instead of
- improving the life of other people whose lives are not in immediate danger?
or
- saving the lives of many people in the future through disease-prevention programmes (such as treating high blood pressure or lowering blood cholesterol levels)?

If the Council considers that NICE should ignore the rule of rescue – why?
    If the Council considers that the rule of rescue should be applied – when?
    And what limits are there?'

In the final analysis, most of the Citizens Council agreed that individuals in desperate and exceptional circumstances should sometimes receive greater help and prioritisation than is justified by a purely utilitarian approach.

A number of reasons were put forward for this, but one of the strongest that came through repeatedly was that this was the mark of a humane society – it was 'our badge of humanity' and in this sense it had a wider significance in terms of 'social capital' than it might seem at first glance.

Quality of life was key to deciding whether to save or prolong life. Indeed some members had shifted to believing that improving the quality of the remaining months of someone with a terminal illness was as important as saving life in the first place.

Members reportedly felt uncomfortable with the tough choices they were being asked to make between competing examples of deservedness. And most of them tried at the beginning of the meeting to circumvent the law of 'opportunity costs', which states that in a world of finite resources, helping one person means that someone else cannot be helped.

Ultimately most Council members agreed that the NHS had a duty to save a life – but not at any cost – and this must depend to some extent on the quality of the life being saved. Where views differed was on whether the 'rule of rescue' – or exceptional case treatment – was an appropriate way of achieving this.

Those who opposed its use, did so on the basis of cost and equity. As one member said: 'You have got to help [patients in immediate danger of dying] but not at the cost of the overall well-being of the population as a whole.'

But the majority felt there would inevitably be exceptional cases where these arguments were overridden by other considerations. In fact it was considered that society as a whole would be diminished if we did not intervene in these situations. 'It cannot always be about cost but about how we care for those in most need with all our resources,' commented one member. Another put it even more simply: 'We must be able to afford our principles.'

Those of the Citizens Council who rejected the rule of rescue altogether, did so believing that all funding decisions had to be made on the basis of the greatest good for the greatest number. They felt this was the only approach that was transparent and equitable, and pointed out that there would always be a long queue of deserving exceptional cases. Once you accepted one of these, you would open the floodgates to everyone seeking exemption and where would that end? 'This is certain financial suicide,' commented one member.

Regardless of which side of the argument members were on, most believed the approach the Council favoured would ensure consistency and fairness. 'We as a cross-section of the public, don't expect to like all the decisions made by NICE; but what we do expect is to know the basis on which these decisions are made.'

SEVENTH CITIZENS COUNCIL REPORT: INEQUALITIES IN HEALTH

On this occasion the Citizens Council was asked to consider which of two broad strategies would be more appropriate for NICE to follow.

Option 1

Is it appropriate for NICE to issue guidance that concentrates resources on improving the health of the whole population (which may mean improvement for all groups) even if there is a risk of widening the gap between the socio-economic groups?

Option 2

Is it appropriate for NICE to issue guidance that concentrates resources on trying to improve the health of the most disadvantaged members of our society, thus narrowing the gap between the least and most disadvantaged, even if this has only a modest impact on the health of the population as a whole?

And for each of these strategies, are there factors that should merit special consideration?

The Citizens Council was unable to reach unanimous agreement. In the end 1 member felt unable to express a firm preference, 10 members backed Option 1, while 15 favoured Option 2. Neither preference was unqualified.

Together with evidence from the tracking questionnaires, this finding indicates that despite many and varied reservations, a majority of the Citizens Council would sympathise with NICE strategies intended not only to improve public health for all, but also to offer particular benefit to the most disadvantaged.

EIGHTH CITIZENS COUNCIL REPORT: ONLY IN RESEARCH

In this meeting, NICE asked the Citizens Council:

'In what circumstances is it justified for NICE to recommend that an intervention is used only in the context of research?'

The Citizens Council presented the circumstances that they thought should be taken into account when NICE considers whether or not to make an 'only-in-research' recommendation (*see* below). Most members felt that all but one of these were uncontentious. Many of their conclusions were unanimous; where there was a division of opinion the voting figures are presented.

NICE should take into account the following:

➤ whether at least one appropriate, relevant study
➤ is planned (e.g. the study will definitely start within six months of the guidance publication date), or
➤ is in progress (e.g. recruitment to the study is open, and is expected to last at least one year beyond the guidance publication date), or
➤ could be established quickly.
➤ whether the question addressed by the study will contribute to reducing the uncertainties identified during the preparation of NICE guidance.
➤ whether the research is feasible (in terms of numbers of patients, recruitment, etc.) and is likely to deliver results within an appropriate time period.
➤ whether the study will be multicentre with broad coverage of the relevant geographical area and population to ensure that as many eligible patients as possible can realistically access the technology within a study setting.

Agree: 21
Disagree: 4
Don't know: 2

➤ whether further research is good value for money.
➤ whether a fully supportive decision would lead to significant irretrievable
   fixed costs of implementation.
➤ whether a fully supportive decision, instead of an 'only-in-research'
   recommendation, would terminate research in progress or prevent new
   research from beginning and thus have a negative impact on the future
   collection of relevant information.
➤ whether it is realistic to hope that research can be carried out to the
   satisfaction of NICE? Factors to be considered include: the timeliness of
   the research; potential number of patients able to participate in research;
   the pace of the current research; the precise nature of the questions to be
   answered.

In addition to this list of 'circumstances' the Council asked to add the
following:
➤ An 'only-in-research' decision should not be used as a way of avoiding the
   need to say 'no' to interventions that are excessively costly.
➤ NICE should resist the attempts of patient groups, the media and other
   bodies that may wish to pressure it into choosing an 'only-in-research'
   decision when a 'no' decision is the more appropriate response.
➤ Patients already receiving a treatment should continue to do so even if that
   treatment is then categorised as 'only in research'.
➤ When making an 'only-in-research' decision NICE should define the
   questions it wants answered through research, and also prescribe the
   methodology to be used.
➤ NICE may wish to consider how 'only in research' could be used as means
   of encouraging innovation.
   Agree: 23
   Disagree: 4
   Don't know: 0
➤ With treatments for life-threatening conditions where there is no other
   remedy available, NICE should consider granting it the 'benefit of the
   doubt' with an 'only-in-research' decision rather than a 'no'.
   Agree: 25
   Disagree: 1
   Don't know: 1
➤ NICE should be mindful of the risk of discriminating against groups
   perceived to have a low quality of life as measured by the QALY
   system.
   Agree: 22
   Disagree: 1
   Don't know: 4

➤ NICE should do what it can to ensure that the research findings are fed back to the clinicians who can benefit from them.
➤ The 'also-in-research' option proposed by one of the speakers should not be adopted.
Agree: 24
Disagree: 2
Don't know: 1

The Citizens Council also wanted NICE to note one other topic on which they voted. By a large majority (24 out of 27 members voting) the Council felt that the assessment of cost effectiveness and the use of the QALY system should be the subject of a future Citizens Council meeting.

NINTH CITIZENS COUNCIL REPORT: PATIENT SAFETY

NICE had been asked by the Department of Health to develop solutions to reduce or prevent harm to patients while under the care of the NHS. At the time NICE intended to take cost effectiveness as well as clinical effectiveness into account when developing patient safety solutions. Therefore the Citizens Council was asked:
➤ Does the Citizens Council accept that it is appropriate when developing 'patient safety solutions' that NICE take the costs, as well as the benefits, into account?
   • If the answer is 'yes,' what principles of cost effectiveness should apply?
   • If the answer is 'no,' what criteria should NICE apply in deciding whether or not it should recommend a particular safety solution to the NHS?

A substantial majority of the Council agreed that it is appropriate for NICE to take account of costs as well as benefits when developing guidelines on the improvement of safety.

They were aware that the methodology currently used by NICE – which is also likely to be used in developing safety solutions – relies on the QALY. However, a substantial majority felt that the QALY methodology did not lend itself well to making decisions on cost effectiveness in the area of patient safety, because the QALY does not include certain costs, such as litigation, cost to carers and those left behind following a death.

However, mindful that the QALY continues to be widely used in work of this kind and that there was no other adequate cost-effectiveness tool available, most of the Citizens Council felt it would not be helpful to NICE simply to dismiss QALYs out of hand. So, in the absence of a suitable alternative, the Council suggested that if NICE was to use QALYs in assessing safety solutions, it did so with a degree of flexibility greater than is normally the case when setting a threshold figure above which expenditure for a particular purpose is judged unacceptable.

While the Citizens Council recognised that departing from a single standard threshold created problems of its own – not least in consistency – it was also aware that NICE did on occasion move outside its own self-imposed limits when particular circumstances seemed to justify such an action.

When asked what circumstances might be relevant when making decisions on the cost of equipment or practices intended to avoid error, the Council envisaged a sliding threshold limit. Factors that might contribute to the case for moving a threshold included:

➤ the severity to an individual of any likely injury or harm resulting from the error

➤ the wider cost to society of coping with the aftermath of the error – cost to those left caring or bereaved, cost of litigation

➤ the extent to which the error is unique to the medical environment – falls can happen anywhere, but only in operating theatres do people have the wrong kidney removed

➤ the possibility that failure to address the safety issue in question could have a severely damaging effect on public confidence in the NHS.

TENTH CITIZENS COUNCIL REPORT: QUALITY-ADJUSTED LIFE YEARS (QALYS) AND THE SEVERITY OF ILLNESS

NICE asked the Citizens Council to consider whether NICE and its advisory bodies should take the severity of a disease into account when making decisions. If yes, should the advisory committees take severity into consideration alongside the cost and clinical-effectiveness evidence, or should severity be included in the calculation of the QALY?

The Citizens Council members concluded, by 24 to 2, that NICE and its advisory bodies should indeed take the severity of a disease into account when making decisions. Among the members who took this view, there was unanimity that rather than do so by including severity in the calculation of the QALY, it should be taken into consideration alongside the cost and clinical effectiveness evidence.

They reached this conclusion mainly because they felt that the process of the QALY calculation already takes some account of severity, and because any changes intended to weight QALYs further in this respect would inevitably make them more complicated and harder to understand, and may also distort the model. This in turn could lessen their transparency, thereby making any attempt to understand a committee's decision more difficult.

The alternative of taking severity into consideration would give appraisal committees more flexibility. The Council said it would not wish to see a mathematical or other formulaic approach to this task as such a step might simply recreate the rigidity of the QALY component of the decision. One suggested course of action was to add something about severity to NICE's statement on social value judgements.

Transparency is vital to the acceptance of NICE decisions, not only in the way that committees reach them, but in how they are subsequently reported and explained. The Council was clear that people must always be able to understand a committee's reasoning.

The Council also felt that there was a problem with the EQ-5D questionnaire used by NICE because it was too blunt to capture all the factors relevant to the definition of a good or bad quality of life. Members said they would prefer an approach that incorporated more of the social as well as the medical model of health and disease. They also wanted an approach that could take more account of the views of those who have first-hand experience of the circumstances being rated, although they appreciated this could be difficult to achieve.

The Council said that they were not calling for the questionnaire or the QALY to be abandoned; rather they were suggesting that, in the light of experience so far, it was time they were subjected to a thoughtful and penetrating review.

ELEVENTH CITIZENS COUNCIL REPORT: DEPARTING FROM THE THRESHOLD

NICE's threshold has always triggered debate and as part of a series of activities to address these concerns, NICE asked the Citizens Council to consider in what circumstances it should recommend interventions where the cost per QALY is above the threshold range of £20 000 to £30 000?

Two of the 29 Council members attending the meeting took the view that there were no circumstances in which NICE appraisal committees should depart from the established threshold. These two members took no further part in the voting.

Of the remaining 27 Council members, the numbers who favoured taking account of a list of various possible circumstances were (in order of support):
➤ the treatment in question is life saving (24)
➤ the illness is a result of NHS negligence (23)
➤ the intervention would prevent more harm in the future (23)
➤ the patients are children (22)
➤ the intervention will have a major impact on the patient's family (22)
➤ the illness is extremely severe (21)
➤ the intervention will encourage more scientific and technical innovation (21)

➤ the illness is rare (20)
➤ there are no alternative therapies available (19)
➤ the intervention will have a major impact on society at large (16)
➤ the patients concerned are socially disadvantaged (13)
➤ the treatment extends life (10)
➤ the condition is time limited (9)
➤ the illness is a result of corporate negligence (2)
➤ the stakeholders happen to be highly persuasive. (0)

TWELFTH CITIZENS COUNCIL REPORT: APPRAISING THE VALUE OF INNOVATION AND OTHER BENEFITS

As part of the input into Sir Ian Kennedy's study on how NICE should value innovation[2] the Citizens Council was asked to provide a view on innovation. It was asked to explore which features of innovation should be considered when assessing its value, specifically in the context of healthcare.

Each member of the Citizens Council was asked to choose three features from the list below – final votes are included.
➤ It increases quality of life. (26)
➤ Other innovations may be developed from it in the future. (11)
➤ A large number of people will benefit from it. (10)
➤ It saves your life. (9)
➤ It increases life expectancy. (9)
➤ It meets a previously unmet need. (6)
➤ It prevents a condition. (5)
➤ It cures a condition. (5)
➤ There are few other treatment options. (1)
➤ It reduces risk to the patient. (0)
➤ It has a one-off cost rather than ongoing costs. (0)

The Citizens Council was asked to tackle two other questions. The first was, if the innovation is more expensive than NICE's current cost per QALY gained threshold and does not demonstrate benefits at the moment but could well do so in the future, what should NICE do?

Fifteen of the Citizens Council members thought that NICE should say 'no' for the present, and ask the developers to fund and carry out more research themselves. The remaining 13 members also wanted NICE to say 'no' for the present but preferred that further research be co-funded for the developers on condition that the public would get a return proportionate to any investment.

For a clearer insight into these conclusions the Citizens Council was asked more specifically who should bear the costs and risks of research and development. Members were presented with five choices:

➤ the developer
➤ the NHS
➤ the taxpayer
➤ charities
➤ joint sharing between taxpayer and developer.

Seventeen members felt that the developer of the technology should bear the full cost. The rest opted for joint sharing between the taxpayer and the developer.

The Citizens Council also offered NICE a number of suggestions (listed in the body of the report)[3] on how it might improve its communication with the public about innovation.

REFERENCES

1 National Institute for Health and Clinical Excellence. *Reports*. London: NIHCE. Available at: www.nice.org.uk/getinvolved/patientandpublicinvolvement/opportunitiestogetinvolved/citizenscouncil/reports/reports.jsp (accessed 22 September 2009).
2 National Institute for Health and Clinical Excellence. *Kennedy Study of Valuing Innovation*. London: NIHCE. Available at: www.nice.org.uk/aboutnice/howwework/researchanddevelopment/KennedyStudyOfValuingInnovation.jsp (accessed 22 September 2009).
3 National Institute for Health and Clinical Excellence. *Citizens Council report: innovation, with invitation to comment*. London: NIHCE. Available at: www.nice.org.uk/getinvolved/patientandpublicinvolvement/opportunitiestogetinvolved/citizenscouncil/reports/reports.jsp?domedia=1&mid=D1838937–19B9-E0B5-D496CA8CE0607B66 (accessed 22 September 2009).

CHAPTER 12

Social value judgements: implementing the Citizens Council reports

Peter Littlejohns and Michael Rawlins

INTRODUCTION

This chapter describes the principles that NICE requires all its advisory bodies to follow when applying social value judgements to the development of all forms of guidance. It is particularly concerned with the social value judgements that NICE should adopt when making decisions about effectiveness and cost effectiveness. The principles are intended for three audiences:

➤ NICE's advisory bodies responsible for developing individual items of NICE guidance

➤ those involved in designing or revising the processes for developing NICE guidance

➤ NICE's stakeholders and the wider public, to enable them to understand the social values that underpin NICE guidance.

Who has developed these principles?

The principles are unusual in being the direct responsibility of NICE's Board. However, although the Board is ultimately responsible for all NICE guidance, the content of individual forms of guidance is usually approved on its behalf by senior members of staff.

The first edition of these principles[1] was prepared using

➤ the published literature

➤ reports by NICE's Citizens Council

➤ results of a survey conducted on behalf of NICE.

This second edition was prepared using:

➤ further reports from the Citizens Council[2-6]
➤ comments on the Citizens Council reports by NICE's technical staff
➤ publications commenting on the first edition of *Social Value Judgements*
➤ a survey of NICE's advisory body members on how the principles set out
  in the first edition of *Social Value Judgements* had been used and how they
  could be improved
➤ a report from a roundtable discussion that explored the principles in the
  first edition in relation to contemporary bioethics and political philosophy
➤ a consultative workshop on social value judgements involving NICE staff,
  its advisory bodies and outside experts
➤ legislation on human rights, discrimination and equality as reflected in
  NICE's equality scheme.

Outline of the chapter
We begin by discussing ethical principles that relate to healthcare decisions and
how decisions can be made. We set out the fundamental principles that underlie
NICE and its processes and how these are applied when developing guidance.
We then explain how NICE responds to comments and criticisms before describing how NICE aims to avoid discrimination and promote equality. We finally
describe the particular considerations that apply to public health guidance and
look briefly at reducing inequalities before discussing how NICE should follow
these principles.

PRINCIPLES OF BIOETHICS
Moral principles
NICE subscribes to widely accepted moral principles that underpin clinical and
public health practice.[7-12] These so-called 'four principles' have been adopted by
NICE because they provide a simple, accessible and culturally neutral approach
that encompasses most of the moral issues that arise in healthcare.[13] NICE recognises that there are tensions both within and between these principles; and it
accepts that no one principle has an overriding priority. Indeed these guidelines
are, to a considerable extent, concerned with attempting to resolve the inherent
tensions between them within the context of the social value judgements that
NICE and its advisory bodies have to make. The principles are as follows.

➤ Respect for autonomy. This recognises the rights of individuals to make
  informed choices about healthcare, health promotion and health
  protection. The concept of 'patient choice' arises from this principle.
  It cannot, however, be applied universally or regardless of other social
  values. For example, some people may be unable to make informed
  choices because of mental or physical incapacity, and some public health

measures must be imposed on whole populations (such as smoking bans in enclosed spaces).

➤ Non-maleficence. The second principle involves an obligation to not inflict harm (either physical or psychological) and is associated with the maxim 'first, do no harm'. As any treatment or intervention can potentially have adverse consequences, it may be necessary to balance the benefits and harms when deciding whether an intervention is appropriate.

➤ Beneficence. This is closely related to non-maleficence and involves an obligation to benefit individuals. But no clinical or public health intervention is always beneficial for everyone. In the context of the work of NICE, it is the balancing of benefits and harms that is usually more relevant.

➤ Distributive justice. The final principle is concerned with providing services in a fair and appropriate manner. This is a particular problem in healthcare because of the inevitable mismatch between demands and resources. This leads to the problem of 'distributive justice', or how to allocate limited healthcare resources fairly within society.

➤ There are, broadly, two approaches that can be taken to resolve such problems in publicly funded healthcare systems.

➤ The utilitarian approach involves allocating resources to maximise the health of the community as a whole. It allows an efficient distribution of resources, but sometimes at the expense of fairness. It can allow the interests of minorities to be overridden by the majority; and it may not help in eradicating health inequalities.

➤ The egalitarian approach involves distributing healthcare resources to allow each individual to have a fair share of the opportunities available, as far as is possible. It allows an adequate but not necessarily maximum level of healthcare, but raises questions as to what is 'fair'. An egalitarian approach cannot be fully applied when there are limits on resources.

➤ There is no consensus as to which approach provides the more ethical basis for allocating resources.[7,13,14] Each has strengths and weaknesses, and NICE does not subscribe fully to either approach. Rather, NICE seeks to apply the principles that underpin the NHS through an emphasis on 'procedural justice' (*see* 'Procedural justice' below).[14] This focuses on ensuring that the processes by which healthcare decisions are reached are transparent, and that the reasons for the decisions are explicit. It does not attempt to resolve the conflicts between these different approaches.

Procedural justice

Procedural justice provides for 'accountability for reasonableness'. The processes decision-makers use to make their decisions must have four characteristics: publicity; relevance; challenge and revision; and regulation.[14] These are described further by Professor Norman Daniels in Chapter 15.

It is particularly important for NICE to be 'accountable for its reasonableness' because it provides advice to the NHS. As the NHS is funded from general taxation, it is right that UK citizens have the opportunity to be involved in decisions about how the NHS's limited resources should be allocated.

The following describes the features of the processes relating to procedural justice that are used to develop NICE guidance.

FUNDAMENTAL OPERATING PRINCIPLES

There are both legal obligations and fundamental principles underlying the processes by which NICE produces its guidance and these must be adhered to.

Legal obligations

NICE is bound by its Establishment Order,[15] Directions from the Secretary of State for Health,[16] and legislation on human rights, discrimination and equality.

NICE's Establishment Order[15]

'Subject to and in accordance with such Directions as the Secretary of State may give, the Institute shall perform –

(a) such functions in connection with the promotion of clinical excellence, and the effective use of available resources in the health service

(b) such functions in connection with the promotion of excellence in public health provision and promotion and in that connection the effective use of resources available in the health service and other available public funds

(c) such other functions as the Secretary of State may direct'.

Secretary of State's Directions to NICE[16]

The Secretary of State's Directions to NICE require that (among other matters) in the appraisal of the clinical benefits and the costs of interventions, NICE should consider the following factors:

(a) the broad balance of clinical benefits and costs

(b) the degree of clinical need of patients with the condition or disease under consideration

(c) any guidance issued to the NHS by the Secretary of State that is specifically drawn to the attention of NICE by the Secretary of State and any guidance issued by the Secretary of State

(d) the potential for long-term benefits to the NHS of innovation.

The Secretary of State's Directions limit the interventional-procedures programme to considerations of safety and efficacy.

NICE is committed to promoting equality, eliminating unlawful discrimination and actively considering the implications of its guidance for human rights. It therefore aims to comply fully with legislation on human rights, discrimination and equality. NICE's *Equality Scheme and Action Plan 2007–2010* describes in detail how it meets these commitments and fulfils its obligations.[17]

Assessing the impact of its guidance on equality is now an integral part of NICE's guidance development process. All guidance centres record the impact of equality issues at all stages of the guidance development. NICE also tries to involve the widest possible range of organisations that are concerned with inequality in developing its guidance. NICE uses public consultation to seek a diverse range of views on the potential impact of guidance on equality.

Procedural principles

Although each type of NICE guidance is developed using a different process, all these processes follow the same procedural principles. They therefore share common features as described below.

Scientific rigour

NICE's guidance development processes should be scientifically rigorous. Guidance should be based on a systematic review of the relevant published literature as well as, when appropriate, unpublished literature.

Inclusiveness

The development of NICE guidance should include all parties with a legitimate interest in the guidance. This includes relevant professional bodies, patients and patient–carer organisations, health-related industries and the wider public health community. All parties should be involved in determining the scope of the guidance at the start of the development process, and have an opportunity to comment on drafts of the guidance.

Transparency

NICE publishes descriptions of all its guidance development processes to ensure that its work is as transparent as reasonably possible. Most evidence supporting its recommendations is published. Only in exceptional circumstances does NICE accept unpublished evidence that must remain 'confidential' to protect the commercial or academic interests of a company or organisation. Initial and final drafts of all forms of guidance are published, and interested parties may comment even if they are not registered as stakeholders or consultees. NICE guidance explains the reasons for the advice and the way NICE has interpreted the available evidence.

Independence

All NICE guidance is developed by members of its independent advisory bodies. The members of these bodies are drawn from the NHS, academia, individuals with experience of the relevant industries and patient–carer organisations. All members have to declare any relevant interests both annually and at each meeting they attend.

Challenge

All four guidance programmes allow consultees and stakeholders to comment on drafts of guidance. In the technology appraisals programme, consultees have rights of appeal to a panel appointed by NICE's Board and all appeals are open to the public. The interventional procedures programme has a resolution process. Because NICE is a public body, its guidance can also be challenged in the courts.

Review

The need to review NICE guidance is assessed between three and four years after publication. This may happen sooner if significant new information becomes available.

Support for implementation

In 2004, NICE launched an implementation strategy to support the uptake of its guidance. It aims to ensure that there are mechanisms for implementing guidance recommendations as part of quality improvement throughout the NHS and partner organisations.

Timeliness

Parliament, the public, patients and the NHS expect NICE to publish guidance in a timely manner. But the desire to rapidly develop guidance sometimes conflicts with the need for guidance to be based on robust evidence and subject to appropriate consultation. Appropriate arrangements are required for guidance to be developed at the time it is needed without compromising its quality.

All these features relate to the procedural justice requirement for 'accountability for reasonableness' described above. They give legitimacy to NICE guidance, and therefore should also apply to any future forms of guidance.

EVIDENCE-BASED DECISION MAKING

NICE guidance is evidence based. NICE assesses the clinical, public health and cost effectiveness of interventions before deciding whether and how to recommend their use. NICE applies the following principles when developing evidence-based guidance.

Clinical and public health effectiveness

Principle 1

NICE should not recommend an intervention (a treatment, procedure, action or programme) if there is no evidence, or not enough evidence, on which to make a clear decision. But NICE's advisory bodies may recommend the use of the intervention within a research programme if this will provide more information about its effectiveness, safety or cost.

NICE expects its advisory bodies to use their scientific and clinical judgement to decide whether the available evidence is sufficient to provide a basis for recommending or rejecting particular clinical or public health measures. NICE recognises, however, that there is a difference between 'evidence of lack of effectiveness' and 'lack of evidence of effectiveness'. In general, therefore, NICE's advisory bodies should avoid recommending interventions where evidence of their effectiveness is absent or too weak for reasonable conclusions to be drawn.

NICE's advisory bodies may sometimes recommend that an intervention is used only within a research programme. If this is the case, the advisory body should consider whether the intervention is reasonably likely to benefit patients and the public, how easily the research can be set up or whether it is already planned or in progress, how likely the research is to provide further evidence, and whether the research is good value for money.

Cost effectiveness

Principle 2

Those developing clinical guidelines, technology appraisals or public health guidance must take into account the relative costs and benefits of interventions (their 'cost effectiveness') when deciding whether or not to recommend them.

Except in the case of interventional procedures, NICE and its advisory bodies have to consider whether interventions are cost effective before recommending their use in the NHS.

Deciding which treatments to recommend involves balancing the needs and wishes of individuals and the groups representing them, against those of the wider population. This sometimes means treatments are not recommended because they do not provide sufficient benefit to justify their cost.

NICE's interventional procedures guidance does not address cost effectiveness; therefore, principles 3 and 4 below do not apply to it.

Assessing cost effectiveness

> **Principle 3**
>
> Decisions about whether to recommend interventions should not be based on evidence of their relative costs and benefits alone. NICE must consider other factors when developing its guidance, including the need to distribute health resources in the fairest way within society as a whole.

NICE assesses how cost effective an intervention is by comparing its cost against the gain in health outcome (benefit) it is expected to provide. This is known as cost-utility analysis. The main health outcome measure that NICE uses is the quality-adjusted life year (QALY) – *see* 'Glossary' for a definition.

NICE uses the QALY as an outcome measure because it takes into account not only the increased life expectancy from an intervention, but also the quality of the increased life. It reflects the value judgement that mere survival is an insufficient measure of benefit; and that the expected quality of life years gained also needs to be considered. The QALY also provides a 'common currency' that allows different interventions to be compared for different conditions. This allows NICE to make its decisions consistently, transparently and fairly. Cost-utility analysis cannot, however, be the sole basis for NICE's decisions and NICE expects its advisory bodies to use their judgement when considering the results of cost-effectiveness analyses.

Comparing the cost effectiveness of different interventions

> **Principle 4**
>
> NICE usually expresses the cost effectiveness of an intervention as the 'cost (in £) per quality-adjusted life year (QALY) gained.' NICE should explain its reasons when it decides that an intervention with an incremental cost-effectiveness ratio (ICER) below £20 000 per QALY gained is not cost effective; and when an intervention with an ICER of more than £20 000 to £30 000 per QALY gained is cost effective.

Where one intervention appears to be more effective than another, NICE must decide whether the increased cost, associated with the increased effectiveness, represents reasonable 'value for money' for the NHS. NICE generally compares interventions by calculating the incremental cost-effectiveness ratio (ICER). ICERs are expressed as cost (in £) per QALY gained.

NICE has never identified an ICER above which interventions should not be recommended and below which they should. However, in general, interventions with an ICER of less than £20 000 per QALY gained are considered to be cost effective. Where advisory bodies consider that particular interventions with an ICER of less than £20 000 per QALY gained should not be provided by the NHS they should provide explicit reasons (e.g. that there are significant limitations to applying the evidence for effectiveness to the population as a whole). Above a most plausible ICER of £20 000 per QALY gained, judgements about the acceptability of the intervention as an effective use of NHS resources will specifically take account of the following factors.

➤ The degree of certainty around the ICER. In particular, advisory bodies will be more cautious about recommending a technology when they are less certain about the ICERs presented in the cost-effectiveness analysis.

➤ Strong reasons that indicate the assessment of the change in the quality of life has been inadequately captured and may therefore misrepresent the health gain.

➤ The intervention is an innovation that adds demonstrable and distinct substantial benefits that may not have been adequately captured in the measurement of health gain.

As the ICER of an intervention increases in the £20 000 to £30 000 range, an advisory body's judgement about its acceptability as an effective use of NHS resources should make explicit reference to the relevant factors considered above. Above a most plausible ICER of £30 000 per QALY gained, advisory bodies will need to make an increasingly stronger case for supporting the intervention.

Individual choice

Principle 5

Although NICE accepts that individual NHS users expect to receive treatments to which their condition will respond, this should not impose a requirement on NICE's advisory bodies to recommend interventions that are not cost effective enough to provide the best value to users of the NHS as a whole.

The Citizens Council emphasised the importance of individual choice and of respecting individuals' values, cultural attitudes and religious views. However, it recognised that it might sometimes be necessary to limit individual choice in the interests of the population as a whole.

Although NICE agrees that respect for autonomy and individual choice are important for the NHS and its users, this should not mean that NHS users as a whole are disadvantaged by guidance that recommends interventions that are not clinically and/or cost effective.

Rare conditions

NICE considers that it should evaluate orphan drugs to treat rare conditions in the same way as any other treatment. It does not expect to receive referrals from the Secretary of State for Health to evaluate ultra-orphan drugs (drugs used to treat very rare diseases or conditions) because the Department of Health has other mechanisms to assess the availability these drugs.

Rule of rescue

There is a powerful human impulse, known as the 'rule of rescue', to attempt to help an identifiable person whose life is in danger, no matter how much it costs. When there are limited resources for healthcare, applying the 'rule of rescue' may mean that other people will not be able to have the care or treatment they need.

NICE recognises that when it is making its decisions it should consider the needs of present and future patients of the NHS who are anonymous and who do not necessarily have people to argue their case. NICE considers that the principles provided in this document are appropriate to resolve the tension between the needs of an individual patient and the needs of present and future users of the NHS. Therefore NICE has not adopted an additional 'rule of rescue'.

RESPONDING TO COMMENTS AND CRITICISM

Principle 6

NICE should consider and respond to comments it receives about its draft guidance, and make changes where appropriate. But NICE and its advisory bodies must use their own judgement to ensure that what they recommend is cost effective and takes account of the need to distribute health resources in the fairest way within society as a whole.

NICE's processes encourage the active involvement of consultees and stakeholders. It is the duty of NICE and its advisory bodies to consider and respond objectively to their comments and, where appropriate, to amend its guidance.

Sometimes attempts are made, directly or indirectly, to influence NICE's decisions in ways that are not in the broad public interest. While NICE must consider all relevant comments, it alone must make the decisions entrusted to it. NICE and its advisory bodies must not respond to 'special pleading'. NICE should be consistent in using its own judgement to make sure that what it recommends is cost effective and takes account of the need to distribute health resources in the fairest way within society as a whole.

AVOIDING DISCRIMINATION AND PROMOTING EQUALITY

The NHS aims to provide free, necessary and appropriate treatment to the UK population. Legislation on human rights, discrimination and equality requires that patients' access to NHS care is not blocked or hindered because of their race, disability, age, sex/gender, sexual orientation, religion, beliefs or socioeconomic status. NICE's Board expects everyone working for or with NICE to be particularly vigilant to avoid discrimination and to promote equality.

NICE's general approach to equality was discussed above. This section deals with circumstances that demand NICE to restrict an intervention to a particular group of people within the population.

Race (ethnicity)

NICE should recommend the use of an intervention for a particular ethnic group only where there is clear evidence of difference in its clinical effectiveness within such a group that cannot be identified in any other way.

Disability

NICE should take special account of the needs of disabled people. This includes considering whether there are obstacles that might prevent them from benefiting from NICE guidance. Where necessary and appropriate it should deliberately take account of these needs.

Age

There is much debate over whether, or how, age should be taken into account when allocating healthcare resources. The Citizens Council considered that health should not be valued more highly in some age groups than in others and that social roles at different ages should not affect decisions about cost effectiveness. However, it said that where age is an indicator of benefit or risk, it can be taken into account.

NICE's general principle is that patients should not be denied or have restricted access to NHS treatment simply because of their age. NICE guidance should refer to age only when one or more of the following apply.

➤ There is evidence that age is a good indicator for some aspect of patients' health status and/or the likelihood of adverse effects of the treatment.

➤ There is no practical way of identifying patients other than by their age (for example, there is no test available to measure their state of health in another way).

➤ There is good evidence, or good grounds for believing, that because of their age patients will respond differently to the treatment in question.

If NICE and its advisory bodies refer to age in guidance, the guidance should include an explanation of their reasons.

Sex/gender and sexual orientation

In making recommendations, NICE and its advisory bodies should avoid distinguishing between individuals on the basis of their gender or sexual orientation unless these are indicators for the benefits or risks of interventions.

Conditions associated with stigma

Some conditions, such as sexually transmitted diseases and drug dependency are associated with stigma. NICE does not consider that stigma itself is a reason for altering its normal approach to assessing cost effectiveness. However, NICE is aware that stigma may affect people's behaviour in a way that changes the effectiveness of an intervention. It also recognises that the relief of stigma may not always be captured by routine quality-of-life assessments. Therefore, NICE expects its advisory bodies to take these considerations into account.

Behaviour-dependent conditions

The Citizens Council advised that NICE should not take into consideration whether or not a particular condition was self-induced. Receiving NHS care should not depend on whether people 'deserve' it or not.

NICE should not produce guidance that results in care being denied to patients with conditions that are, or may have been, dependent on their behaviour. However, if the behaviour is likely to continue and can make a treatment less clinically effective or cost effective, then it may be appropriate to take this into account.

Socioeconomic status

Principle 7

NICE can recommend that the use of an intervention is restricted to a particular group of people within the population (e.g. people under or over a certain age, or women only), but only in certain circumstances. There must be clear evidence about the increased effectiveness of the intervention in this subgroup, or other reasons relating to fairness for society as a whole or a legal requirement to act in this way.

NICE should not recommend interventions on the basis of individuals' income, social class or position in life. Nor should individuals' social roles at different ages affect decisions about cost effectiveness.

PARTICULAR ISSUES FOR NICE GUIDANCE ON PUBLIC HEALTH

Public health initiatives make a major contribution to promoting good health and preventing ill health. The broad moral principles set out in this chapter apply equally to the development of both NICE's clinical guidance and its public health guidance. The requirements of 'accountability for reasonableness' described fully in Chapter 15 also apply to public health guidance.

However, 'public health' refers to the efforts of society as a whole to improve health. Interventions are aimed at prevention rather than treatment; and at populations rather than individual patients. This raises additional ethical problems.[18] Traditional bioethics emphasises the freedom of the individual, but to be successful, a public health approach may, as in the case of seat-belt legislation, limit individual autonomy.

NICE asked the Citizens Council to consider when it is legitimate for authorities to intervene in a mandatory way to address a public health problem. The Council considered that non-mandatory public health measures, such as providing education and information, were preferable to mandatory ones, provided they were effective. Non-mandatory measures were less controversial and easier to introduce, and did not breach the principle of individual autonomy. In many cases, non-mandatory measures are the only practicable way of improving public health (e.g. safe sex, taking exercise and attending smoking cessation clinics). However, although the Citizens Council thought that where possible people should have freedom of choice and be responsible for their own health, they also considered that, when necessary, NICE should recommend that interventions should be mandatory.

NICE should take the following issues into account when deciding whether to recommend that a measure is mandatory.

➤ The balance of benefits and costs. In the case of a national emergency, the evidence needed to justify a public health intervention might be of lower quality.
➤ The importance of respecting individual choice but within limits.
➤ The proportionality of the measures relevant to the risk.
➤ The requirement to reduce health inequalities.
➤ Potential adverse effects on vulnerable members of society.
➤ The need to ensure mandatory measures are monitored, evaluated and (as required) discontinued so as to avoid harmful consequences.
➤ The importance of implementing measures in consultation with the broader community and after explaining the reasons for their introduction.

This approach is compatible with the stewardship model described in the Nuffield Council on Bioethics report.[18] However, implementing mandatory public health measures is the responsibility of the Government and not that of NICE.

REDUCING HEALTH INEQUALITIES

Principle 8

When choosing guidance topics, developing guidance and supporting those who put its guidance into practice, NICE should actively consider reducing health inequalities including those associated with sex, age, race, disability and socioeconomic status.

While the overall health of the population continues to improve, the differences in health between the rich and poor have increased despite many attempts to change this. NICE asked the Citizens Council to consider NICE's approach to health inequalities.

The Citizens Council concluded that, where feasible, NICE should support strategies that improve the health of the population while offering particular benefit to the most disadvantaged. The Council believed this would help to reduce health inequalities, particularly in the context of public health.

The Board considers that NICE has a duty to take into account the impact of its guidance on health inequalities; and that its advisory bodies should try to ensure that implementing NICE guidance will not widen existing inequalities. Furthermore, in promoting measures to reduce health inequalities, NICE's Board places particular emphasis on the importance of selecting the right topics on which to develop guidance; and in supporting those with the responsibility for putting NICE guidance into practice.

FOLLOWING THE PRINCIPLES

NICE must follow the principles described in this chapter if its guidance is to meet the legal and moral obligations to the people it serves. Together the principles fulfil the requirements of 'accountability for reasonableness'.

NICE's Board believes a statement of broad compliance with the principles should be included in all NICE guidance as well as in its process and methods manuals. In situations where guidance appears to depart from these principles, it should be stated with a clear explanation. NICE has a responsibility to monitor adherence to and ensure compliance with these principles, particularly those relating to legislation on human rights, discrimination and equality.

REFERENCES

1 National Institute for Health and Clinical Excellence. *Social Value Judgements: principles for the development of NICE guidance.* London: NIHCE; 2005. Available at: www.nice.org. uk/media/873/2F/SocialValueJudgementsDec05.pdf (accessed 22 September 2009).

2 National Institute for Health and Clinical Excellence. *NICE Citizens Council Report: mandatory public health measures.* London: NIHCE; 2005. Available at: www.nice.org. uk/nicemedia/pdf/NICE_Citizens_Council_Report_Public_Health.pdf (accessed 22 September 2009).

3 National Institute for Health and Clinical Excellence. *Report of the Citizens Council: rule of rescue.* London: NIHCE; 2006. Available at: www.nice.org.uk/nicemedia/pdf/Rule_of_rescue_report_final_0606.pdf (accessed 22 September 2009).

4 National Institute for Health and Clinical Excellence. *Report of the Citizens Council: inequalities in health.* London: NIHCE; 2006. Available at: www.nice.org.uk/nicemedia/pdf/CCreportonHealthInequalities.pdf (accessed 22 September 2009).

5 National Institute for Health and Clinical Excellence. *Report of the Citizens Council: only in research.* London: NIHCE; 2007. Available at: www.nice.org.uk/media/129/29/OIRReport300407.pdf (accessed 22 September 2009).

6 National Institute for Health and Clinical Excellence. *Report of the Citizens Council: patient safety.* London: NIHCE; 2007. Available at: www.nice.org.uk/media/A3E/37/CCPatientSafetyReportJune07V1.0.pdf (accessed 22 September 2009).

7 Beauchamp TL, Childress JF. *Principles of Biomedical Ethics.* 5th ed. Oxford and New York: Oxford University Press; 2001.

8 Gillon R. *Philosophical Medical Ethics.* Chichester: Wiley; 1985.

9 Gillon R. *Principles of Health Care Ethics.* Chichester: Wiley; 1994.

10 Beauchamp TL. The 'four principles' approach. In: Gillon R, editor. *Principles of Health Care Ethics.* Chichester: Wiley; 1994. pp. 3–12.

11 Gillon R. The four principles revisited. In: Gillon R, editor. *Principles of Health Care Ethics.* Chichester: Wiley; 1994. pp. 319–34.

12 Gillon R. Medical ethics: four principles plus attention to scope. *BMJ.* 1994; **309**: 184–8.

13 Cookson R, Dolan P. Principles of justice in health care rationing. *J Med Ethics.* 2000; 26: 323–9.

14 Daniels N, Sabin JE. *Setting Limits Fairly: can we learn to share medical resources?* New York, NY: Oxford University Press; 2002.

15 *Statutory Instrument 2005 No. 497. The National Institute for Clinical Excellence (Establishment and Constitution) Amendment Order 2005.* London: Her Majesty's Stationery Office.

16 Department of Health. *Directions and Consolidating Directions to the National Institute for Health and Clinical Excellence.* London: Department of Health; 2005. Available at: www.dh.gov.uk/en/Publicationsandstatistics/Publications/PublicationsLegislation/DH_4109216 (accessed 22 September 2009).

17 National Institute for Health and Clinical Excellence. *NICE's Equality Scheme.* London: NIHCE. Available at: www.nice.org.uk/aboutnice/howwework/NICEEqualityScheme.jsp (accessed 22 September 2009).

18 Nuffield Council on Bioethics. *Public Health: ethical issues.* London: Nuffield Council on Bioethics; November 2007.

CHAPTER 13

The view of a Citizens Council member

Brian Brown

It is not often that a Lord and principal of an Oxford College shares a platform with a Harvard Professor of Ethics and a plumber, but that is what happened at the session on 'Making social value judgements' at the 2007 NICE annual conference.

Lord Krebs had chaired the working group that produced the Nuffield Council on Bioethics report, *Public Health: ethical issues,*[1] and Norman Daniels discussed his work on meeting health needs fairly and how judgements should be made (*see* Chapter 15). I was a plumber and member of the Citizens Council.

I had the pleasure of being a member of the NICE Citizens Council from its beginning in November 2002 until I retired in June 2006. I attended eight meetings during this time.

The concept of the Citizens Council is that 30 members of the public, not involved in the healthcare system, meet to debate topics about social values. I should stress that we have never been asked to comment on any specific treatment or intervention. Those decisions fall outside the role of the Citizens Council.

An independent company is responsible for the administration of the Citizens Council and the selection of members. It also organises and conducts the actual meetings. This helps to ensure that there is a visible element of independence between NICE and the Citizens Council. However, this independence caused some problems at the beginning. For the first few meetings NICE largely kept away. This meant that as we challenged the topics and sought to understand what was being asked of us, the facilitators had no way of checking if we were on the right path. Now, whilst the meetings are still conducted independently, they are held at NICE headquarters. This allows NICE to observe the Council and gives the facilitators easy access to iron out any problems. The lesson here is that because we are discussing questions for NICE, we cannot be totally independent from them.

The 30 members of the Citizens Council are selected to reasonably reflect the geographic, demographic and ethnic nature of England and Wales. One-third of the Council membership is replaced each year. This idea was not received well at first. We had formed strong bonds during the first three meetings as we had all learnt how to deal with the topics, with NICE, and with each other. We all wanted to keep the group together for a pre-set period and then replace all members at once.

We lost that fight, but nevertheless my experience of two changes of members has been very positive. It helped to prevent members from becoming 'institutionalised', that is, too much a part of NICE instead of being totally independent, and ensured that fresh perspectives were regularly introduced. It also helped to constantly challenge individuals' pre-set views. It has kept the pot boiling.

We discussed a range of topics during my time on the Citizens Council ranging from clinical need to health inequalities. A topic that resulted in a particularly lively discussion was whether the NHS should pay premium prices for ultra-orphan drugs. This involved paying many times over the accepted NICE definition of cost effectiveness for treatments of very rare conditions. The debate centred on whether a treatment had to be provided just because it was available, irrespective of the disproportionate cost to the local primary care trust. It was no surprise that the views of the members ranged from 'yes, pay whatever it takes to treat people' to 'no, if it is outside the accepted definition of cost effective, don't provide the treatment'.

In a case like this there is no way that a consensus view can be reached; the opinions are too far apart. The best that can be done is to debate the topic fully to allow everyone to get a full understanding of the consequences of their individual decision on both the people with the conditions and on the rest of the population. Indeed part of the debate was to list the consequences of each decision, both positive and negative. This helped many people to reach their decision. The final report in this case could say only that so many were in favour of one option and so many in favour of the other. What the report could do, however, was give a sense of what influenced people to hold their particular views and demonstrate that other factors had been considered. The report also detailed a tracking survey, which was conducted at various times throughout the meeting. This showed how opinion had moved during the course of the three days of discussion. On this occasion the only common ground was that these conditions should be centrally funded, although we acknowledged that even this was not a complete solution, and caused other problems.

The Citizens Council report is posted on the NICE website for comment from all interested parties. The report is then presented to the NICE Board at one of its regular public meetings. This allows both the report and the public's comments on it to be considered by NICE. Therefore, what you get from the

Citizens Council is informed, questioned and reasoned opinion rather than an off-the-cuff 'this is what I think'.

THE IMPORTANCE OF GAINING PUBLIC PERSPECTIVE

The topics we discussed in the Citizens Council are not ones that have clear logical answers – otherwise we would not be required. Instead, they usually involve the conflict between what we would like to do, and what we can afford to do. Which groups can we afford to treat and which can we not? Are there any exceptions, and why? What information do we provide and what do we withhold?

We were no more qualified to judge these issues than health professionals. Indeed on most occasions we were quite daunted by the complexity of the questions we were asked. We were, by design, just 30 ordinary people off the street. However we were no *less* qualified to judge the issues than health professionals. That is because the issues affect us all – how we behave as a society and how our money is to be spent by the NHS.

NICE sets guidelines for which interventions should be available in the NHS and these decisions are often not a simple case of 'this one is affordable whereas this one is not'. In some cases there are added pressures like an intervention being expensive but it is for children – is it still justifiable? Or an intervention for an ultra-orphan disease – is that a special case? The panels making the decisions have to make judgements that are not as clearly defined as the more technical aspects of the issue, such as cost and efficacy.

NICE decisions are open to challenge and it is important for NICE to be able to defend its methods and practices. This was clearly seen earlier this year with the judicial review into the Alzheimer's ruling.[2] The Citizens Council is I think, largely a means of demonstrating that NICE is taking public perspectives into account. It provides some extra validation of NICE decisions and is a part of the transparent way NICE works.

It should be said that from the beginning we were very much an experiment in public involvement, indeed for the first four meetings we were the subject of an Open University study. All our proceedings were videoed and recorded and it was quite eerie at first. There was a very steep learning curve for all sides: the members, the facilitators and NICE. Even now I think NICE is wrestling with exactly what to do with the output from the Citizens Council.

I remember attending a NICE Board meeting where the future of the Citizens Council was being discussed. One member who was obviously opposed to the concept of a Citizens Council said: 'I told you what you would get, some would say this and some would say that'. That is indeed what you do get. What you also get is some insight into why people have the values they have.

What have I learnt about making social value judgements? The biggest lesson I have learnt is that there is no right or wrong answer.

There are people who will not accept the reality of limited funds. Given a hard choice, some people cannot or will not make it. Their answer is always to throw more money at the problem. This raises questions about the extent to which we allow public involvement in decision making. There are people in the NHS making some really difficult decisions, such as primary care trust commissioners. One commissioner who came to speak to us at the Council would quite welcome a judicial review of funding to establish 'right' from 'wrong'. At the moment all her decisions are open to question.

Another point I have learnt in the process is to beware of the power of the 'last speaker'. When the Council discussed age, there were some very powerful presentations from both sides and I remember my opinion swaying backwards and forwards after each speaker. It was only in the cool peace of the evening that I could put it all together and make a reasoned decision that I could justify.

I also observed that medical science is moving faster than society's capacity to use it. Many new treatments are very expensive to implement. Should we use them?

Many of the problems affecting the NHS are not strictly health issues but are symptoms of a wider problem in society, such as obesity, smoking and drugs. The NHS has to deal with the symptoms, but society should be dealing with the causes. There is a modern tendency to put responsibility on to the state rather than accept personal responsibility. It is quite clearly a personal decision to put food into your mouth or light a cigarette. The outcome must surely be a personal responsibility. Yet these are major problems for the NHS and society.

Finally let me say that I would rather social value judgement decisions were made in forums like the Citizens Council than on the basis of opinion polls collected on street corners. After receiving the questions for meetings, I have discussed the issues with family and colleagues at work. Many of the responses I got were the off-the-cuff, 'gut feel' kind. An example would be age. Most people would say that children should get preferential treatment and extra spending. When it came to the meeting however, this was rejected. The majority felt that positive discrimination was still discrimination. Later when I discussed that decision with the same people back at home, they were quite sympathetic with the outcome and understood the reasoning behind it. I was and remain quite proud of that decision.

REFERENCES

1 Nuffield Council on Bioethics. *Public Health: ethical issues.* London: Nuffield Council on Bioethics; 2007. www.nuffieldbioethics.org/fileLibrary/pdf/Public_health_-_ethical_issues.pdf (accessed 22 September 2009).

2 National Institute for Health and Clinical Excellence. *Alzheimer's Judicial Review.* London: NIHCE. Available at: www.nice.org.uk/newsroom/factsheets/alzheimersjudicialreview.jsp (accessed 22 September 2009).

CHAPTER 14

A Citizens Council in the making: dilemmas for citizens and their hosts

Celia Davies, Margaret Wetherell and Elizabeth Barnett

I will start this chapter with a question: how feasible is it to call upon ordinary people to come forward and take part in decision making, not just locally, but in relation to the institutions of central government?[1,2]

There have been numerous citizen participation initiatives in recent years, using citizen juries, peoples' panels, consultative forums and other techniques. They have sought to engage in political debate both already-organised stakeholders and those directly affected by the outcome of an issue. There are fewer examples of new institutions that recruit citizens without an immediate personal interest in an issue, and observe how they work as a group, how they handle complex information and what arguments they find persuasive.

It was this latter kind of participation (involving people with no personal interest or association with a topic) that NICE had in mind when in Autumn 2002, it invited 30 members of the public to form its first 'Citizens Council'.

As a new and inclusive style of organisation, NICE had sought to engage multiple stakeholders from the outset. Its appraisal committees often invited patient groups to evaluate the effectiveness and efficiency of clinical interventions that directly affected them, and NICE acknowledged life experience as a legitimate source of evidence. Its Partners Council regularly met to consider strategy and discuss annual reports. The idea of a Citizens Council represented a novel addition. Would it be possible to explore the value of decisions involving members of the public who had no immediate stake in the outcome of specific enquiries?

Two key questions were uppermost in the minds of some of those closest to the new venture. First, would 'ordinary people' have not only the willingness but also the capacity to debate the complex issues at stake and to form helpful decisions? Second, would it be possible (while hosting meetings, providing information and support) for NICE to avoid the charge of 'citizen capture'?

An independent evaluation team was recruited to observe and record the proceedings of the Council over its first two years and to track the kinds of dialogue that took place. On the basis of what is probably still the most sustained and detailed ethnographic study to date, what can be concluded about the vexed questions of citizen capacity and capture?[2] What messages can be gleaned about citizen-participation initiatives of this kind; are they fashion, fantasy or feasible?

The first part of this chapter concentrates on citizens themselves, on what they bring to such an arena and how they interact once there. Later, the focus turns to the matter of hosting and designing citizen participation, and what may be learnt from the very active attempts made by the host organisation not only to encourage and shape the deliberations of the Council itself, but also to position the results in relation to its many – not always enthusiastic – stakeholders. The chapter considers seven messages relating to the twin questions of 'citizen competence' and 'citizen capture'. It emphasises the need to actively foster citizen potential in order to help the councillors produce a report that can be used by NICE in the complex daily process of developing guidance.

> **Message 1:** Despite widespread assumptions about citizen apathy, it is possible to encourage large numbers of people to come forward for membership of a citizens' assembly.

NICE received around 35 000 expressions of interest in a Citizens Council and over 4000 people followed through with an application – and all responded to a challenge not about their own local services, but about improving the NHS as a whole. What prompted them to act?

Among the 30 people selected, wanting to make a contribution, helping to improve things and a conviction that the public should be more involved in the services they funded and used, were the main reasons cited for wanting to join the Council. Comments such as these implied a concept of active responsibility as a citizen. Hoping to be stretched, to test themselves and to do something new, formed another cluster of reported motivators. What became apparent in the evaluation study was a sense of an unused resource among citizens, of a hunger to learn and of a willingness to enter a collective arena which, many admitted with some trepidation, was something quite outside their previous experience. Hopes that they would 'make a difference' and 'improve the NHS' were not fulfilled during the period we studied the Citizens Council, but the enthusiasm of virtually all the members remained apparent throughout. Two years on, their assessments remained largely positive and a substantial number of the original citizen members even had plans to do more in future and to get involved in their local health trusts, for example.

Much of the credit for the high level of interest in this particular citizen-participation initiative must be attributed to the host organisation and the external team it recruited to support and facilitate members of the Council. NICE was able to orchestrate substantial high-profile media attention. This work was complemented with active networking by facilitators already experienced in working with excluded groups. Public debate often portrays modern citizens as individualistic, cynical and disaffected or apathetic. The experience of NICE lends support to arguments that the public are not necessarily apathetic and uninterested in political participation for the public good.[3]

> **Message 2:** When asking citizens to thoughtfully consider strategic issues of policy direction, clarifying the grounds on which they are being asked to speak is fundamental. This includes creating (jointly with them) an 'expertise space' in which they can call upon familiar and emerging speaking positions.

Coming forward to participate as individuals is one thing. Pulling off collective, and specifically deliberative, participation – a form of discussion that will tease out different positions, explore conflicting rationales for action and share ideas about what might constitute the common good – is another. Although the amount of deliberation that took place in the Citizens Council increased over time and across the meetings observed, the amount remained very small. Over the first two years of the Citizens Council, hopes for a high-quality deliberative debate were not met.

Political scientists interested in the potential for participative and deliberative democracy have sometimes claimed that the central dilemma here is that of overcoming self-interest. Data from the Citizens Council suggested that it was not so much a question of whether people could transcend self-interest, but of actively creating an expertise space for citizens as citizens – a firm base on which to engage with each other and with the questions set. In principle, Council members had a diversity of experiences to bring to the matters under discussion. In practice, bringing personal experience into the debate was fraught with difficulty. Coming as 'ordinary people', just what could they bring?

An analysis of transcribed exchanges showed that Council members were far more precarious with *their* contributions based on 'common sense', a 'down to earth' or 'bigger picture' view than with those of the professionals. Citizens experimented with various speaking positions – the interrogator, for example, or the student. Different styles and speaking positions jostled with each other as citizens sought to find ways of making their interactions meaningful and relevant. In the process, focused questioning of witnesses, sustained discussion of their contributions and the exploration of potentially diverse positions in relation to the topic, were casualties.

Compounding this difficulty was the sheer unfamiliarity of the situation, and the potential conflicts it might generate. Council members had expressed concerns in initial interviews not only about what would be required of them, but about how they would get on with each other, and how they would deal with any disagreements and conflicts that arose. The pressure, certainly at the outset, was to move quickly to consensus rather than engage in the more risky pursuit of naming and exploring their differences. Posing highly abstract questions for discussion, as NICE had done, exacerbated the difficulties.

> **Message 3:** Deliberation is a resource-intensive activity that needs continuing and imaginative forms of nurture, both by citizens and their hosts, to create an expertise space in which citizens feel comfortable to contribute.

A great deal changed over the first four meetings, as hosts and facilitators worked to find ways that would engage citizens more effectively. Different styles of presenting and of assimilating information were tried as well as ways to explore the members' positions on values. Role plays, and teasing out priorities by allocating paper money to photographed individuals, for example, were devices that were light hearted and fun. These were also safe devices for starting to name and explore differences of values. The facilitators made efforts to redesign sessions, incorporating feedback from Council members and moving away from a sole reliance on the formal witness presentations, small groups and plenary debates on which the initial session had relied. This was appreciated by Council members. Less visible was a considerable amount of behind-the-scenes support by facilitators for members, both during the meetings and between them. We tracked differences in emotional tone as this paid off. Council members began to make new sense of the task on which they had embarked, and to enjoy the challenge, not only of making up one's mind, but also of being able to legitimately change it. Familiarity, experience and experimentation with session design all served to enhance the potential for deliberative forms of interaction. Deliberation in the meetings of the Citizens Council, however, continued to occur in a fragile and fitful way.

On reading the early reports of proceedings (prepared by the facilitators and checked with members), critics began to suggest that seemingly high costs could be saved by cutting back on facilitation. As evaluators, our conclusion was the opposite. Facilitating for inclusion – ensuring individuals are heard and that quieter voices find a space – is one thing. Facilitating for deliberation – encouraging the respectful pursuit of a line of thought, allowing constructive challenge, reflection and reviewing – is quite another. And without continuing attention to these matters there is a risk of reinstating the very orthodoxy of thinking that deliberation seeks to disrupt.

> **Message 4:** Citizens are likely to find it difficult to challenge each other's views; they need spaces and social practices that acknowledge and legitimate oppositional ideas in order to embark on an effective deliberative discussion.

Deliberation aspires to bring a significant diversity of positions on a topic into a discussion arena and to give each of these a real chance to find expression. Only if this is done, and if the different positions are understood, acknowledged and explored, can the discussion then move on to consider what might be proposed as the common good. I have already noted Council members' initial hesitancy about expressing their differences. Where a different view counters the conventionally accepted, majority understanding of an issue, there is not only the risk of voicing such a view (that will be queried), but the challenge of finding words with which to articulate it that are both satisfying to oneself and accessible to others. Without ready access to languages of critique, opposition and resistance, or without the easy facility to translate those into accessible terms for others, members may be silenced and the rationale of deliberation put in jeopardy. John Dryzek, prominent political theorist in this field, emphasises that enabling oppositional discourse is pivotal; the whole project of deliberative democracy is to 'retrieve the critical voice'.[4]

A key problem was that readily accessible ideas, received wisdom and orthodox ways of thinking set barriers to the expression of Dryzek's 'critical voice'. One of the most challenging findings of the ethnographic study was an absence of resistance to the ruling point of view and hence of inclusive discussions that might be genuinely oppositional and generative of new ideas. A lack of clarity about the grounds on which citizens could legitimately speak, and pressures to not generate conflict, meant that while differences of class, ethnicity, gender, disability and age were visible to all, these identities were not able to be explored with regard to the topic under discussion. This was borne out in a dramatic incident where members dismissed any notion that such discrimination could be positive and strongly affirmed a call for treating everyone 'the same', at which point the Council burst into applause. Two members sat silent and were clearly baffled by this. A third, who had taken part, noted this and in a later interview mused 'were so many of us wrong?'

A similar incident occurred when the Council concluded that avoiding accusations of ageism simply meant identical treatment for all and this very quickly became a key and uncontested thread in the two meetings on the topic of age. It had the effect of denying the chance to explore fundamental issues in the debate. Later there were efforts on the part of the organisers to devote a session to confronting notions of potential racism and sexism as a way of opening up space for more diversity of voices. This resulted in unease and anxiety. The need for it was questioned and resisted by the majority.

Citizens rarely felt representative of the gender, ethnicity, sexuality class and disability groups to which they belonged. And if they did do so, they did not feel that they could, with ease, represent distinctive counterpositions that such groups might hold. All too often, these dilemmas contributed to a ready – but potentially misrepresentative – homogenising of viewpoints and a restatement of the very orthodoxy of thinking that deliberation seeks to disrupt. A further problem here was that Council members often persuaded each other that personal experience, and the anecdotes that could often bring arguments alive, were somehow not the proper business of the public discourse in which they were engaged. However, in contrast, anecdotes from experts and hosts tended to be appreciated and positively affirmed for their value.

> **Message 5:** Citizens cannot be relied upon to provide the sole source of oppositional ideas; different kinds and levels of critique need to be opened up as part of the process.

How might 'safe spaces' for dialogue across difference be constructed? More thought needs to be given in the academic literature to the subtleties of oppression, the unconscious traces of hegemonic thinking that citizens themselves are likely to bring to the arena (influenced, for example, by the mass media), as well as to the unintended and unacknowledged bias that hosts introduce in the framing of questions. Also, the design of sessions and the choice of witnesses should be considered.

In this case study, as experience developed there were glimpses of facilitative practices that began to open up oppositional possibilities through the identity play that took place when Council members, instead of being expected to give their own views immediately, or to respond to differently positioned experts, were asked to perform set-piece debates on different topics. One of the facilitators in later sessions adopted a 'devil's advocate' role, which appeared to help open citizens' horizons, to challenge them to think differently, to search for alternative formulations and help them tease out implications.

Instances of sustained deliberation took the form of what we called 'collaborative enquiry'. Here the floor is shared by several speakers and the mood is of collective puzzling, all contributing different threads. Speakers finish each other's utterances or end on a question that draws out the next speaker. In this way, the nature of a dilemma and its solution starts to emerge.[1] This offers a style of interaction with the potential to bring new terms into the ways that an official public debate has been cast. But it is not the direct dialogue across difference that is envisaged to generate new policy options and alternatives. What we need to foster, suggests American political scientist Jodi Dean, is not solidarity in sameness but the more difficult solidarity in difference. This demands a pause, respect for the other, and a willingness to reflect aloud and to shift positions.[5] It is useful if the complexity and diversity of personal experience is brought in to harness a process of policy development. But it may not be the only style of interaction that gives deliberation its results. The collaborative power of the social group is all too easily overlooked in a culture that celebrates the rational, individual and combative styles of argumentation. Deliberation may need further development in order to work effectively for citizens.[1]

Be that as it may, deliberative assemblies such as the Citizens Council also need defending for their positions in relation to other, more established and understood, mechanisms of public policy making. The challenge for the host organisation in this case study was not only to find ways of creating deliberation *in situ* in the Council itself – it was also to defend the idea of deliberation and its place in pre-existing organisational arrangements.

Message 6: Deliberation always works in relation to pre-existing relations of power and of accountability; acknowledging this needs to be part of a shared rationale for embarking on it, and to be reflected in the ways in which the outcomes of deliberation are handled.

Advocates say deliberative assemblies will bring new possibilities into the realm of political discussion. Detractors say that such assemblies will be captured – manipulated by the powerful who host them – or they will be cast aside and ignored. Both arguments highlight the question of just what the status of a Citizens Council and its reports and recommendations should be.

At the outset, NICE was mindful of potential criticism surrounding capture and made efforts to step back. An outside team of facilitators was recruited. Senior NICE staff played host at Council meetings and welcomed members, but then left, repeatedly emphasising that their plan was not to influence. And yet, it was NICE who had initiated the process and provided the funding. It was NICE who gave energetic and enthusiastic senior time to a steering group, setting the questions to be explored, naming the witnesses to be called and giving initial consideration to the reports that the facilitators had agreed with members. For the first meeting, and arguably also to some extent for those that followed, the Citizens Council struggled to understand its brief and to find ways to address it. Two discursive worlds had collided. The puzzlement and unease of members was apparent and the result seemed, to the evaluation team, less like capture and more like abandonment. Eventually, it was the outside facilitators, not NICE, who urged that Council members needed to learn more about NICE and to have an initial induction session.

In terms of practical politics, there was no way that the Citizens Council could be an island. NICE was repeatedly faced with a need to 'explain' the Citizens Council to its varied stakeholders. NICE struggled early on, for example, with just where the Council was to fit alongside the already complex consultative processes that constituted its main business.[6] Members of its Partners Council expressed unease, and queried both the potential lack of independence for the citizens and where their views were to fit alongside their own. Board meetings at times meant defending the Council against criticism – often in terms of doubts about value for money. External stakeholder groups were also alert to potential Citizens Council deliberations that might be disadvantageous to them.

Much steering committee time was spent puzzling over the first Citizens Council report and how to interpret and handle it. Council members were invited to attend and present their reports to the Board. Later, a series of impact workshops was put in place to confront the question of just what the options might be for using the results of Citizens Council deliberations (*see* below). And later still, a report was prepared on values, drawing both on Citizens Council reports and other sources. It was clear as the evaluation project ended that the 'join' between the Council and its host organisation was by no means settled. It was still very much evolving.

In summary, a deliberative assembly can have the capacity to disrupt established power relations. Disruption occurs regardless of whether or not its deliberations manage to produce disruptive thinking and regardless too of criticisms that may be levelled at its lack of independence. Deliberative assemblies can be expected to provoke resistance from established groups and the world views they espouse; deliberation's sponsors must expect to actively defend a deliberative assembly against its critics.

> **Message 7:** Integrating a deliberative assembly into established institutional structures entails challenging these very same structures. Creating space to reflect on the alternative possibilities outside established structures is an important step to enable deliberation to be a genuinely generative process.

There will inevitably be a debate surrounding the significance of a deliberative assembly and the fate of its recommendations. This was particularly clear in this case study at the point where NICE initiated its in-house workshops as a means to actively integrate the work of the Citizens Council into its programmes of work, and to consider what was to be done with its outputs. Some participants were very enthusiastic. However, the language of science and its assumptions surrounding acceptable evidence threatened to discredit the Council's output.

How exactly were members selected and could they be said to be representative? Was all relevant information on the table? Were arguments fully tested in debate? Would opinion polling be a preferable device? What, too, of the merits of social science methodologies and techniques for eliciting value choices? Counter-arguments stressed the value of an informed public and the generative potential of dialogue. At times, it was only the strongest steer from the Chair that prevented a group from completely undermining the value of the Council.

Some have concluded that the results from a deliberative process should be binding on those who commission it. Any agreement reached through the imperfect and contingency-laden process that is likely to be deliberation in practice, however, is perhaps better regarded as one resource among others for a democratic decision. Council members themselves seemed to concur with this view. While some did raise concerns that the Council might end up as a 'cosmetic exercise', in the main, they were content to see their views being discussed and being taken into account. Some members, indeed, were distinctly uneasy about the responsibility that would be implied by anything more than this.

There is also a point here about formal lines of political accountability. Developments following the completion of the research were a reminder of the complex and contested political accountabilities in which a host organisation can be enmeshed. NICE was in the news, for example, over pressure to speed up its decision processes, and controversy erupted over the use of the drug trastuzumab (Herceptin). These and similar developments underline the point that deliberative assemblies are always nested in structures of power and authority. Deliberation can give glimpses of alternative possibilities, but these need to be reflected upon, reinforced or challenged in other spaces and places – and meshed with ongoing structures of accountability and decision making.

CONCLUSION

The Citizens Council of NICE was an ambiguous project and full of dilemmas. Its resolution was still being shaped as the study ended. Creating a forum such as the Council – one in which policy ideas can be digested and challenged, consciousness can be expanded and hard choices can be addressed in terms of a notion of the common good – is a dream that continues to inspire politicians, academics and ordinary citizens themselves. Turning the dream into reality entails not only the challenges of creating and nurturing an expertise space for citizens, as discussed earlier in this chapter, but also piloting the very idea of a deliberative assembly between the rocks of organised interests and pre-established mechanisms of accountability.

The Citizens Council of NICE could have died at the end of the first two years; it was still fragile, still under development in terms of how it worked and still in doubt for many of those who needed to be persuaded of its value. That it did not die is testament to the determination, imagination and reflective capacity of all those involved – citizens and their hosts alike.

Acknowledgements

Support from the NHS R&D Methodology Programme for an evaluation study of the Citizens Council is gratefully acknowledged.

REFERENCES

1 Davies C, Wetherell M, Barnett E. *Citizens at the Centre: deliberative participation in healthcare decisions.* Bristol: Policy Press; 2006.
2 Davies C, Wetherell M, Barnett E, *et al. Opening the Box: evaluating the Citizens Council of NICE. Report prepared for the National Coordinating Centre for Research Methodology, NHS Research and Development Programme.* London: Open University; 2005.
3 White I. *Power to the People. The report of POWER: an independent inquiry into Britain's democracy.* York: York Publishing Services; 2006.
4 Dryzek J. *Deliberative Democracy and Beyond: liberals, critics, contestations.* Oxford: Oxford University Press; 2000.
5 Dean J. *The Solidarity of Strangers: feminism after identity politics.* London: University of California Press; 1996.
6 Davies C. Grounding governance in dialogue: discourse, practice and the potential for a new public sector organisational form in Britain. *Public Adm.* 2007; **85**(1): 47–66.

CHAPTER 15

Accountability for reasonableness and the Citizens Council

Norman Daniels

What is the value of NICE's Citizens Council to the decision-making process about new services? In what follows, I shall offer an argument in favour of a deliberative process that incorporates views of the public – a key stakeholder in all NHS decisions. This argument provides a theoretical answer to the question about the added value of the Citizens Council. An important set of research questions, however, can only be answered by examining the Citizens Council's effects on deliberation and the public acceptability of decisions.

I shall begin by noting some of the kinds of social value judgements that arise in the process of NICE advising the NHS. Many of these judgements create reasonable disagreement among people. In fact, I shall claim, we lack consensus on adequate moral principles to resolve many of these disagreements. As a consequence, we should rely on a fair, deliberative process to arrive at decisions that people can regard as fair and legitimate. This is an appeal to a form of procedural justice.

Specifically, I shall describe four conditions that such a process should meet in order to hold decision makers accountable for the 'reasonableness' of their decisions. One of those conditions involves the search for rationales that all – those making the decision and (ideally) those affected by the decision – can agree are relevant. The Citizens Council is a method for improving deliberation in that process and to bring a typical citizen's reflections to bear on the ethical controversies that underlie specific limit-setting decisions. Their deliberations aim to identify what is important to the public and what should be considered in NICE decisions. I shall conclude with what we might hope to learn about the effects of including the Citizens Council in the decision-making process.

SOCIAL VALUE JUDGEMENTS IN NICE ADVICE

NICE uses cost-effectiveness analysis in making recommendations to the NHS about coverage for new technologies. Wisely, NICE sees this as one input into an evidence- and value-based decision. In taking this stance, it is in agreement with the recommendation of the public health service panel on cost-effectiveness analysis and with a recent Institute of Medicine report on its use in regulatory contexts.[1,2]

Cost-effectiveness analysis is relevant to decision making because one goal of NICE's policy toward population health is to improve the overall level of health in a population and get the optimum aggregate health benefit. This is measured in quality-adjusted life years (QALY) per pound spent. But this is not the only goal of health policy. Justice also requires that we distribute health benefits fairly in a population – and that idea is not exhausted simply by giving people equal access to covered benefits. Although efficiently promoting population health is one social value, other social values about fairness are in tension with it and reasonable people may disagree about how to weight them. Table 15.1 illustrates this point.

TABLE 15.1: Cost-effectiveness analysis versus fairness (equity).

	Cost-effectiveness analysis	Fairness
Best outcomes versus fair chances	Best outcomes	Weighted chances
Priority to worst off	None	Some – varies
Aggregation	Any	Some

Cost-effectiveness analysis takes an implicit stance on three distributive questions and many people object to the fairness of that stance. First, it always favours choices that produce best outcomes. In doing so, it ignores the objection that this may deny a fair chance to other choices for which outcomes are not as good. There is empirical evidence that many people prefer choices that offer some benefit for a wider number of people. This problem lies at the heart of orphan-drug policy, for example, as treatments for rare conditions will often be less cost effective than treatments for more prevalent conditions.

Cost-effectiveness analysis also takes a controversial position on a second distributive question, namely, how much priority to give to those who are worst off. For the sake of argument, let us consider being sickest to count as being worst off. Cost-effectiveness analysis gives no priority to these patients – a QALY is a QALY to whoever it is delivered and wherever in a lifespan it is delivered. In contrast, most people think it is fair to give some priority to those who are worst off, but they may disagree about how much. If we can do very little for people who are worst off, but we can do significantly more for others not quite so sick, in our example, we may care more about delivering the much greater benefits to the less unwell than the much smaller benefits to the more unwell. Different people will trade these benefits in different ways.

Finally, cost-effectiveness analysis allows aggregation across all health effects and so allows *modest* benefits to *more* people to outweigh *significant* benefits to *few* people. For example, if a way of delivering small benefits (shortening the discomfort of a sore throat by a day) to large numbers produces greater benefit, per pound spent, than saving the lives of a few people, then it prefers the more cost-effective approach. Many people think this violates concerns about fairness, rejecting the idea that collective tiny benefits can compete with saving lives. In short, letting cost-effectiveness analysis be the only guide means taking a contested position on fairness on three key issues.

The best outcomes/fair chances problem, the priorities problem and the aggregation problem also arise when we are concerned with reducing health inequalities – although this is less noticed as an issue. Suppose we identify a health inequality that seems clearly unjust. An example might be race inequalities in health in the US – these are significant and arise at every socioeconomic status level. Some inequalities are the result of different ways a decision is employed – a number of studies have shown that different treatments are offered to black and white people with matched clinical conditions, suggesting some form of stereotyping or discrimination by providers. Suppose we try to reduce the inequality. We will bump into the distributive problems noted before. For example, a strategy of sensitivity training might target the inequality better but not improve the level of population health as much as a strategy aimed at training all providers in the use of clinical guidelines. In short, we can help those who are *unjustly* worse off more, but perhaps only at the expense of not producing as much health benefit in the population as a whole.[3,4]

Other social value judgements are also contested, such as those regarding how age can be taken into account in resource allocation, or those that take responsibility for health into account.[5,6] By saying these judgements are contested, I mean that reasonable people can disagree about them. In addition, we don't have a sufficiently defined consensus on principles to resolve our disagreements on these matters.

FAIR PROCESS AND ACCOUNTABILITY FOR REASONABLENESS

If we lack adequate principles to resolve disagreements about social values, one strategy (besides working harder to find such principles) is to rely on procedural justice to provide fair solutions. Specifically, if we judge a process fair, we may accept its outcomes as fair. This appeal to procedural justice lies behind the emphasis Jim Sabin and I put on developing a fair process for decision making about priority or limit setting in our book, *Setting Limits Fairly:*

can we learn to share medical resources?[7,8] We described four conditions, that we thought were the minimum requirements to arrive at fair and legitimate decisions.

Publicity. The rationale for all decisions must be publicly accessible so that people affected by them understand why choices that fundamentally affect their well-being, were made.

Relevant reasons. The rationale for decisions must be based on reasons that fair-minded people agree are relevant. Fair-minded people are people interested in being able to justify their decisions to each other. Often, a mechanism for vetting such reasons is to involve a broad group of stakeholders in the decision, although the exact form for such involvement may vary considerably with the institutional level at which decisions are made (I discuss the rationale for stakeholder involvement shortly).

Revisability and appeals. Decisions must be evidence- and argument-based – a fair process must allow decisions to be reviewed as new considerations become available. Further, there are often specific groups or individuals who do not quite fit the rules or reasoning underlying some choices and who are unduly burdened by them. Such people need a fair hearing to appeal decisions that deny them fundamental treatments.

Enforcement. There needs to be assurance, often in the form of regulation, which ensures the procedures are ones that comply with the first three conditions.

Together, these conditions make decision makers accountable for the reasonableness of their decisions. The publicity and relevance conditions mean that the public can understand the grounds for these decisions. Over time this will enable a kind of social learning that broadens democratic understanding of these decisions. The public record constitutes a kind of case law that reveals the underlying moral commitments and allows assessment of their coherence over time. The public may still not agree with all decisions but objections may be narrower in scope and not be based on perceptions of unfairness and a lack of moral legitimacy.

THE RATIONALE FOR STAKEHOLDER INVOLVEMENT

How should the relevance of reasons behind decisions be determined? Where possible, stakeholders affected by decisions should be involved in determining which reasons count as relevant. In the case of many decisions made by public agencies, this feature of a fair process is not only feasible but is required as an important aspect of administrative process. For example, US regulatory agencies must subject proposed rules to public comment and hearings. In my earlier characterisation of the legitimacy problem, I urged that we take the perspective of those affected by a decision, including those whose health needs are not met as a result of giving priority to the needs of others. Stakeholder involvement would therefore be one clear way of introducing that perspective. The introduction of the Citizens Council into decision making by NICE in the UK is a recognition of the importance of such an input to public agencies.

For private organisations making limit-setting decisions, such as US health plans or NGOs in developing countries, it may not be possible to expect or require stakeholder participation in the vetting of reasons. However, consumer participation has been strongly advocated by some commentators and is sometimes part of the community outreach effort of NGOs.[9–11] Since we are seeking an account of fair process that can be used across the full range of institutions where limit setting is carried out, it may be necessary to compromise on the issue of stakeholder involvement in these contexts, even if such involvement would clearly improve accountability for reasonableness. A key issue is whether this is a compromise of principle or not. The answer requires us to know what the role of stakeholder involvement is in establishing legitimacy.

Some people intuitively think that consumer or stakeholder participation would contribute to legitimacy directly, and that it is necessary in order for legitimacy to be achieved. There are two central rationales for this view. For the first, consumer participation is necessary for legitimacy because participating consumers *represent* other consumers, or even the public as a whole. Through their representation, the decision-making process is made more democratic. With this rationale, consumer participation contributes to legitimacy through this democratisation of the process.

In the second rationale, consumer participation is seen as a form of *proxy consent*. The participants consent on behalf of all others, and their full involvement in the informed decision acts as a substitute for actual consent by others.

Both of these rationales suffer from the same fatal flaw. In the vast majority of situations there is no plausible sense in which the consumers selected to participate actually represent other consumers in the sense that elected officials represent the public. We have no publicly endorsed mechanisms that establish a selection process as a form of democratic representation and there is no recall authority over the alleged representatives. The closest we come to such representation is when publicly authorised officials, over whom we do exercise democratic control, designate particular consumers to participate. However, the delegated authority granted to these consumer participants does not match that of institutions such as private organisations that make limit-setting decisions – with the very rare exception of organisations with a consumer governance structure like the Group Health Cooperative in Washington State.

The complete absence of any democratic procedure or proxy-selection process weakens claims that consumer participation contributes to legitimacy. This means that consumer participation is not generally either a necessary or a sufficient condition for establishing legitimacy.

Nevertheless, stakeholder participation can increase the legitimacy of limit-setting decisions in both private and public organisations by increasing accountability for reasonableness. Stakeholder participation increases the likelihood that a broader range of relevant reasons and rationales will be aired in the decision-making process. For example, a study of consumer input in a public-sector mental-health managed-care programme showed that consumer participation could highlight issues such as the need for better hospital discharge planning with families and more Spanish language services.[12] Similarly, a study of limit setting in Canada showed that consumers can make a distinctive contribution to cancer policy, provided that there is a critical mass of consumers and provided that they have time to build trust with other members of the decision-making group.[13]

A second way in which consumer participation can enhance accountability for reasonableness is by providing a clear mechanism through which transparency may be achieved. Consumer participants are not sworn to secrecy about their deliberations because accountability for reasonableness itself requires publicity about rationales. Participants become a potentially important vehicle for achieving that publicity.

The key idea behind accountability for reasonableness is that fair-minded people will agree that the reasons underlying a decision are relevant and driven by an aim to meet healthcare needs fairly under reasonable resource constraints. Having a broad range of stakeholders playing the role of fair-minded individuals, especially consumers affected by the decisions, gives more credibility to this goal. This approach also avoids falling into the trap of thinking that every idea held in a diverse society must have its direct representative present in the deliberation. The approach does not pretend, however, that organisationally based deliberation can substitute for broader democratic processes. It can facilitate those processes, by modelling a wider deliberation and by educating the public through making its work transparent, but it is not a substitute for full democratic procedures.

Stakeholder participation is given meaning and direction and helps to legitimise decisions if its goal is to improve accountability for reasonableness. It can do this by enhancing the deliberative process at the point of decision making, by broadening perspectives, by testing rationales for acceptability by fair-minded people, and by helping to convey the transparency the process requires. To the extent that accountability for reasonableness is thus improved by consumer participation, the legitimacy of decisions is enhanced.

In short, my suggestion is that accountability for reasonableness is the guiding aim of stakeholder participation, whether in public or private institutions, and participation increases legitimacy only to the extent that it improves such accountability. Attributing this instrumental role to stakeholder participation may seem inadequate to some, but it gives us a more defendable account of how legitimacy is achieved.

NICE AND SOCIAL VALUE JUDGEMENTS

I have not carried out a careful analysis of NICE's process nor examined specific decisions it has made, but from what I know, NICE has gone a long way toward developing a process that measures up to the standards proposed in accountability for reasonableness. First, the evidence base and rationales for decisions are made public and are based on wide consultation with relevant experts. Second, the NICE process allows decisions to be reviewed in light of new evidence, arguments, and appeals. Third, since NICE is an independent and public agency, the enforcement condition is satisfied. Fourth, the Citizens Council constitutes one model for broad public stakeholder involvement in decision making. Let me concentrate on this issue.

Some years ago, I suggested that NICE should do more to engage with stakeholders from the public in making its judgements about specific cases. Since that time, NICE has implemented a plan to rely on a Citizens Council to deliberate about key social value questions that might arise implicitly or explicitly in the advice NICE gives to the NHS.

In the Citizens Council, a representative sample of citizens hears presentations on aspects of an issue and debates their responses to specific questions about social value issues posed by NICE. Important deliberations have included the role of age as a resource allocation criterion, the relevance of reducing health inequalities as a goal of NICE decisions, and the priority that might be given to those at risk immediately as opposed to others (the rule of rescue). I have been impressed by the quality of the deliberation reported in the official reports, although I wish in some cases the deliberation could have gone further. It is important that the Citizens Council does not simply serve as a focus group substitute for broader surveys about public opinion. Although it is important to be informed about what public opinion will be, opinions are only opinions. It is more important to grasp the reasons and arguments that people make when deliberating about these moral issues. The Citizens Council, at its best, goes well beyond simply surveying opinion. Citizens Council reports generally provide thoughtful reasons for their conclusions, including the specifics of their remaining disagreements.

Nevertheless, it remains an interesting question whether the Citizens Council would arrive at similar answers if it were being compelled to participate in specific decisions about interventions, rather than on more general principles or policies that might govern these decisions. A general discussion of social values needs to be tested to see if it really reflects the views people have in more specific decisions. We are interested in the moral commitments revealed by rationales for specific decisions and not just in the general expression of social values in response to more abstract questions. I am not claiming there is a discrepancy, but I would like to determine the relationship between the conclusions of the Citizens Council as now constituted and the decisions Citizens Council members would agree to, were they actually involved in more specific, real decisions about coverage. That is an experiment worth running, although it would be exhausting for participants.

NICE has not simply established the Citizens Council as a public window dressing for what they would otherwise do anyway. In the document *Social Value Judgements: principles for the development of NICE guidance*, NICE articulates principles that should govern its advice for the NHS, and these principles embody conclusions, where available, from Citizens Council deliberations about specific issues.[14]

One of my earlier comments about the distributive complexity of reducing health inequalities bears on a central issue on which the Citizens Council was asked to comment. The Council was asked if NICE's clinical guidance should be weighted to favour the reduction of health inequalities by socioeconomic status, for example by giving more priority to lower socioeconomic status groups. As a result of that Citizens Council deliberation, NICE's statement of principles about social value judgements rejects such a bias in clinical contexts but recommends that public health interventions should aim to reduce health inequalities in socioeconomic status. The problem I earlier pointed to is that reasonable people will continue to disagree about how to balance reductions in socioeconomic status health inequalities with aggregate gains in population health. That is exactly the kind of deliberation about a specific case – with evidence at hand about the trade-offs that would be projected for a public health intervention – that I would want to see Citizens Council debate. It would be interesting to learn if there were more-specific moral rationales (for what trade-offs were allowable) than the general advice embodied in the Citizens Council recommendation. The general advice leaves my concern unaddressed.

It would be useful to develop some empirical evidence demonstrating that the Citizens Council contributes to the perceived legitimacy and fairness of NICE recommendations. Gathering that kind of evidence would require careful research by social scientists who would have to study the attitudes of the public and of providers toward the decisions that NICE makes. It would also be useful to study ways of supporting participants in the Citizens Council without distorting their deliberations. For example, do they learn to behave in ways that are too much modelled on what NICE proposes? It is one thing to argue theoretically about the importance of stakeholder involvement. It is another to understand how to achieve proper deliberation on the part of such stakeholders, and quite another to measure the consequences of including them in the process as a whole.

REFERENCES

1 Gold MR, Siegel JE, Russell LB, *et al. Cost-Effectiveness in Health and Medicine.* New York, NY: Oxford University Press; 1996.

2 Miller W, Robinson LA, Lawrence RS. *Valuing Health for Regulatory Cost-Effectiveness Analysis.* Washington, DC: National Academies Press; 2006.

3 Daniels N. Equity and population health: toward a broader bioethics agenda. *Hastings Cent Rep.* 2006; **36**(4): 22–35.

4 Daniels N. *Just Health: meeting health needs fairly.* New York, NY: Cambridge University Press; 2008.

5 Daniels N. Justice between adjacent generations: further thoughts. *J Polit Theory.* 2008; (in press).

6 Daniels N. Social and individual responsibility for health. In: Knight C, Stemplowska Z, editors. *Distributive Justice and Responsibility.* Oxford and New York, NY: Oxford University Press; 2009.

7 Daniels N, Sabin JE. *Setting Limits Fairly: can we learn to share medical resources?* New York, NY: Oxford University Press; 2002.

8 Daniels N, Sabin JE. *Setting Limits Fairly: can we learn to share medical resources?* 2nd ed. New York, NY: Oxford University Press; 2008.

9 Emanuel E. *The Ends of Human Life: medical ethics in a liberal polity.* Cambridge, MA: Harvard University Press; 1992.

10 Emanuel E. Review of setting limits fairly: can we learn to share medical resources? *N Engl J Med.* 2002; **347**: 953–4.

11 Rodwin M. The neglected remedy: strengthening consumer voice in managed care. *Am Prospect.* 1997; **34**: 45–50.

12 Sabin JE, Daniels N. Public-sector managed behavioural health care: III. meaningful consumer and family participation. *Psychiatr Serv.* 1999; **50**: 883–5.

13 Singer PA, Martin DK, Giacomini M, *et al.* Priority setting for new technologies in medicine: a qualitative case study. *BMJ.* 2000; **321**: 1316–18.

14 National Institute for Health and Clinical Excellence. *Social Value Judgements: principles for the development of NICE guidance.* 2nd ed. London: NIHCE; 2008. Available at: www.nice.org.uk/media/C18/30/SVJ2PUBLICATION2008.pdf (accessed 22 September 2009).

CHAPTER 16

Engaging the American public in setting healthcare priorities

Marthe Gold

Despite a stinging recession accompanied by rising unemployment, healthcare continues to increase the bite it takes from the US economy. At $7290 per capita, Americans spend roughly two times more of their gross domestic product on healthcare than Great Britain[1] while leaving 18% of their population uninsured.[2] US expenditures per capita dwarf those of even the highest spending of industrialised nations, but health outcomes here, as measured by health status and mortality rates, are not as good.[3-5]

Although healthcare reform is the highest domestic priority of the current administration, there are many challenges in finding a strategy that will bring together a fragmented system that has been sustained by massive outlays of both private and public dollars. In a 2007 report, the Congressional Budget Office estimated that private spending on health insurance together with out-of-pocket payments constituted 54.5% of national expenditure on health. Medicaid (18.7%) and Medicare (18.4%), together with other publicly funded programmes, constituted the remaining 45.5%.[6]

Medicaid is a jointly funded (federal–state) means-tested programme that provides healthcare cover for approximately 61 million beneficiaries, roughly half of whom are children of low-income families. Elderly and disabled individuals, who constitute one-quarter of its beneficiaries, are responsible for two-thirds of Medicaid spending, much of it rising from financing long-term care. Medicare is the programme that all Americans eventually become eligible for by reason of age (65 and older) or disability; it is solely federally funded and most like the national health programs of many industrialised nations. Part A of Medicare, or 'Hospital Insurance' is financed through a payroll tax and covers inpatient, skilled nursing and hospice care. Part B, or 'Supplementary Medical Insurance' covers physicians and other healthcare providers, outpatient care, laboratories and medical equipment and is jointly funded by premiums paid by its beneficiaries and through general tax revenues. Part D is a programme to subsidise the costs of prescription drugs. Approximately one-quarter of the costs for the prescription drug benefit, added in 2006, come from enrollee premiums.

Recently trustees for the Medicare programme reported that without increases in taxes to workers and employers, the payroll- and employer-supported Hospital Insurance fund (Part A) will be exhausted by 2017.[7] Parts B and D are expected to remain solvent, in part because their financing is tied to automatic increases in premiums that fall directly on beneficiaries. In 2003, an average of 22% of the income of non-institutionalised Medicare beneficiaries was spent on healthcare, up from 18% in 1999.[8] The current economic climate makes it unlikely that enrollees will be able to continue to meet these increases.

COST CONTROL AND HEALTHCARE REFORM

A number of strategies have been advanced in an effort to control the growth of public and private spending in healthcare. One that has been implemented both by private insurance and by Medicare is to increase the number of 'deductibles' and 'co-pays'. For example, the Medicare prescription drug plan has an initial $295 deductible that patients must pay out of pocket before Medicare provides reimbursement. Once out-of-pocket spending reaches $295, Medicare pays 75% of the bill and patients co-pay until prescription costs reach a 'doughnut hole' – a coverage gap between $2700 and $6154 where all medication expenses are out of pocket.[9] Once the $6154 'catastrophic' threshold is reached, Medicare pays 95% of expenses.

High deductibles and the coverage gap have been shown to place a dispro-portionate burden on sicker people of modest means. Individuals who have illnesses for which there is effective and relatively inexpensive treatment, for example, diabetes or high blood pressure, will often fail to fill prescriptions that are known to prevent serious and expensive complications.[10] Controlling costs by holding patients responsible for first dollar expenses is intended to curtail unnecessary healthcare, but it is a strategy that has been shown to limit non-discretional care as well.

More recently, attention has focused on decreasing unnecessary and inap-propriate care as a means of controlling healthcare spending. Cataloguing of regional variations in medical procedures over the last two decades, by John Wennberg, suggests that limiting healthcare to treatment and interventions that are supported by a scientific evidence base, could substantially decrease the use of health resources in the US.[11–14] Academic medicine and a widening circle of the policy community have called for greater investments in 'comparative effectiveness' research where different strategies for diagnosis and treatment are compared back-to-back. Many believe that ferreting out unnecessary care will substantially control the cost problem and at the same time will improve health outcomes. Opposition to the 'comparative effectiveness' approach has come from quarters that view this as the slippery slope that inevitably leads to using cost-effectiveness analysis (CEA) as a method for determining coverage of services.[15-17]

CEA compares the financial cost of various treatments used in creating a health improvement. Improvements in health are typically calculated in quality-adjusted life years (QALYs).[18] CEA records the 'value' of a treatment by both its effectiveness and its efficiency in creating health, per dollar spent. Medical care can be compared both within and across disease and treatment categories.

While detractors from CEA see it as a harbinger of rationing, others view it as an appealing method for cost control because it informs decisions at the level of coverage policy, without respect to peoples' abilities to meet co-pays and deductibles, and without regard to their underlying health status. For this reason, many view setting priorities at a macro level, rather than at the level of the individual, as a more equitable stance for coverage policy. Although affluent consumers might still choose to buy selected services that were at the margins of effectiveness or cost effectiveness, care that was demonstrably effective and efficient would be available to everyone.

A number of industrialised nations, including Canada, Australia and the Netherlands, use CEA as a component of pharmaceutical coverage decisions, and others, such as New Zealand and the UK, use it more broadly in considering new technologies and resource-intensive technologies.[1-8,19-22] The UK's National Institute for Health and Clinical Excellence (NICE) sets standards and reviews technologies and procedures for use within the healthcare system. NICE issues 'appraisals' of drugs and other treatments based on effectiveness and cost effectiveness. When a favourable appraisal is issued, the NHS must make the service available in all localities within a three-month period. When an appraisal is unfavourable, localities have NICE's official approval to deny cover.[23] Although unfavourable coverage decisions by NICE have sparked controversy and debate,[24] a survey conducted for NICE suggested that the public supports the need for efficiency within the healthcare system.[25]

CEA IN COVERAGE POLICY: NOT (MUCH) IN AMERICA?

In the US there is a widespread perception that the public will never accept economic analyses as a component of healthcare evaluation. The Medicare program, established in 1965, offers a useful window into the debate around CEA. In 1989 the Health Care Financing Administration (HCFA) (now the Centers for Medicare and Medicaid) drafted a regulation proposing that cost effectiveness be added as a criterion in Medicare-coverage decisions. The proposal underwent a decade of internal debate and external vetting before being withdrawn in 1999. Fearing that the use of CEA would diminish their markets, the resistance of the medical device industry was fierce. Both congressional representatives and disease-advocacy organisations rallied against CEA, and arguments were framed that the public would not stand for rationing.[26,27]

Statements by Medicare officials underscored the perceived political vulnerability associated with incorporating economic criteria into coverage decisions. In 1997, Bruce Vladeck, then Administrator of HCFA testified before Congress that CEA raised 'fears of rationing', and would not be used by the agency for coverage decisions.[19,26,28]

In recent years, as CEA methods have become better harmonised and concerns about their potential for bias have diminished, economists and health policy analysts have increasingly called for the use of CEA in healthcare decision making.[18,26,29–33] A *New England Journal of Medicine* article for example, advocated using CEA as one criterion to inform Medicare-coverage decisions.[27] In response, Sean Tunis, then Director of the Office of Clinical Standards and Quality at the federal Centers for Medicare and Medicaid, said: 'Using CEA . . . implies that a clinical benefit will not be available because of cost, which is considerably more difficult to justify than a decision not to provide a service because the risks are expected to outweigh the benefits.'[34]

Attempts to prioritise healthcare services on the basis of their cost effectiveness have also run aground within the Medicaid programme. Oregon's explicit use of CEA methods in its request for a federal waiver to extend Medicaid coverage more broadly for uninsured Oregonians was overturned in part by an argument successfully mounted by the disability community. The community argued that Oregon's methods systematically devalued the lives of disabled Americans.[35] Resistance to use of CEA in the private sector, including the Kaiser Permanente managed care setting[36] and within the Blue Cross Blue Shield Technology Evaluation Center, has also been documented.[37]

There is limited use of CEA in certain US settings. Both the Department of Veterans Affairs[38,39] and the Department of Defense[40] use CEA to make formulary-coverage decisions, and cost-effectiveness information has supplemented guideline development and technology assessment related to preventive services, within the Medicare program.[41] Although WellPoint, a private plan, has been using CEA to begin to inform their formulary-listing process[42] this is a minority position in the private sector. These limited examples are the exceptions that prove the rule of the widespread resistance CEA has encountered within the US.

EMPIRICAL EVIDENCE THAT AMERICANS ARE WILLING TO SET PRIORITIES FOR HEALTHCARE SERVICES

The American public's aversion to 'rationing' has been a widely invoked theme over the past two decades.[43] Political wariness notwithstanding, empirical work that has examined the public's attitudes toward priority setting in healthcare services and use of cost-effectiveness analysis tells a more nuanced tale. What do we actually know?

The Oregon Health Services Commission's (OHSC) attempt to expand health insurance in the early 1990s remains unique in its efforts to solicit public opinion on placing priorities on health service coverage within a publicly funded program. The OHSC sought a waiver from HCFA to make coverage determinations for its Medicaid programme on the basis of the cost effectiveness of a rank-ordered list of treatment/condition pairs that would be funded until the yearly State budget gave out. The Commission used public meetings as forums to solicit the views of Oregonians on the types of services that should be given priority for Medicaid coverage, whatever their cost-effectiveness ratio. Based on these discussions, certain life saving, palliative and preventive care services were moved up on the list.

This natural experiment explored the views of Oregonians about the categories of service to be given priority, but it avoided asking the public head-on questions about ethical or normative views about allocating funds based on efficiency. The explicit focus on 'rationing' (albeit specific to low-income groups) resulted in high-profile media cover of the process, but there was no systematic exploration of public views toward cost-effectiveness analysis and the underlying issues it raises.[44–46]

In an effort to more systematically assess public values and preferences for coverage priorities in public and private insurance programs, researchers developed an exercise called 'Choosing Health Plans All Together' (CHAT).[47] In a sample of 29 Minnesotan citizen groups recruited through employers and community organisations, all said they would trade individual benefits in order to insure the State's uninsured children. The majority were also willing to trade benefits so that uninsured adults could be covered.[48,49] Low-income uninsured individuals in North Carolina were able to use the CHAT exercise to place priorities on the type of services they wished to see insured in comparably priced benefit packages. In groups comprised exclusively of Medicare beneficiaries, participants used the CHAT exercise to make decisions to construct 'more tightly managed' benefit packages. They were willing to forego investigational therapies so that pharmacy, dental and long-term care could be included and additional priority could be placed on insuring the uninsured. CHAT has also informed Medicaid and other discussions in states including Oklahoma, North Dakota and Montana.[50] The focus of this work has been on what services should be covered, rather than explicit explorations of 'whether' and 'for whom' priorities should be set.[49]

Sacramento Healthcare Decisions (SHCD) focused directly on public attitudes toward CEA. It examined the views of members of the California public toward trade-offs between cost and coverage.[51,52] The majority of participants stated that they would accept the use of cost effectiveness by a patient's physician as a criterion for assessing treatment options, but having such judgements made by insurers raised concerns for them. The use of CEA to determine which benefits are covered in a public programme was not explicitly addressed.

SHCD also conducted 27 citizen discussion groups in northern California. Participants were asked to assume the role of members of a National Health Benefits Committee charged with making decisions about whether to cover three medical interventions under consideration by a federally supported programme similar to Medicare. The study sought to understand whether participants would view some treatments as too expensive for the benefit they provided and whether the 'value' (defined as the relationship between cost and benefit) of new procedures and drugs was a relevant consideration for coverage decision making. The interventions, of differing effectiveness, varied from life saving, to those that improved quality of life, to preventive. For each, approximately one-third of participants were unequivocal in their views that the service should be covered. After the discussion, SHCD conducted a survey to ask participants for their views on whether the government should use cost effectiveness in making decisions about what health insurance should pay for. Fifty-one per cent of participants felt it was appropriate to use for most situations and 29% felt it should be used in some, but not routinely.[53]

The views of a New York-based sample were also explored.[54] A diverse group of citizens recruited from the New York County Jury pool were informed about and discussed healthcare costs, CEA methods and common ethical issues embedded in CEA including 'fair innings', 'rule of rescue', trade-offs between length of life and quality of life and the role of individual responsibility.[55–58] At a first meeting, participants received information about the effectiveness of 14 condition/treatment pairs:

➤ treatment for erectile dysfunction
➤ physician counselling for smoking
➤ total hip replacement
➤ outreach for flu and pneumonia
➤ treatment of major depression
➤ gastric bypass surgery
➤ treatment for osteoporosis
➤ screening for colon cancer
➤ implantable cardioverter defibrillator
➤ lung-volume reduction surgery
➤ tight control of diabetes
➤ treating elevated cholesterol

➤ resuscitation after in-hospital cardiac arrest
➤ left ventricular assist device.

A number of these had proved controversial in the discussions of the Medicare Coverage Advisory Committee (MCAC), an expert group that makes coverage recommendations for the Center for Medicare and Medicaid.

Participants were asked to assume the role of 'social decision maker' and prioritise the coverage of these treatments under assumptions of a limited Medicare budget. At a second meeting of the group, participants received information on the cost effectiveness of the 14 treatments and were then asked to review and discuss their rankings.

Providing cost-effectiveness information significantly influenced participant coverage priorities in the direction of favouring more-cost-efficient services. At the conclusion of the focus-group meetings 75% of participants felt 'somewhat' or 'very' comfortable with the use of CEA to inform Medicare coverage of new treatments; 10% said it should 'never' be used. Participants were also asked if they agreed or disagreed that 'people like you' should serve on an independent commission charged by Medicare with making rationing decisions about healthcare; 83% said they agreed.

A similarly configured exercise was conducted in California with six different groups comprised of decision makers (regulators, private and public insurers, and purchasers). Participants ranked the same 14 conditions and accompanying treatments on their priority for coverage, and then, when provided with cost-effectiveness information, re-ranked the interventions in an order that more closely aligned with CEA ratios. A recurrent theme emerging in discussions that followed was the participants' desire that Centers for Medicare and Medicaid Services (CMS) begin to use CEA within the Medicare programs. Many pointed to Medicare's historical leadership in creating changes that rippled through both public and private insurance systems. Follow-up surveys revealed that over 90% of participants felt that CEA should be used as an input to Medicare coverage decisions and that 75% of participants supported its use in private insurance plans.[59]

Although investigations exploring public views on resource allocation are limited, the cumulative evidence supports the idea that members of the public and local decision makers are both able and willing to engage questions about what types of services and what populations should be given priority for insurance coverage.

TIPTOEING AROUND COST EFFECTIVENESS TRADE-OFFS IN DISCUSSIONS WITH THE PUBLIC

Town hall meetings and other community discussion groups have been growing in popularity as a means to engage Americans in the thorny issue of healthcare reform. The Citizen's Healthcare Working Group, a 14-member panel appointed by President Bush in response to a provision of the Medicare Modernisation act of 2003 was charged with developing a framework for a nationwide public discussion about improving the US healthcare system. Congressional statute required that Americans be asked four central questions, one of which was: 'What trade-offs are the American public willing to make in either benefits or financing to ensure access to affordable, high-quality healthcare coverage and services?' The group's final report, presented in Autumn 2006, was based on community meetings in 28 states and responses to internet and paper surveys. A total of 14 165 people were sampled. The Working Group concluded that Americans were able to 'accept limits if based on good medical evidence.' Seventy-five per cent of respondents agreed or were neutral with respect to the statement that health plans should not have to pay for high-cost technologies or treatments that have not been proven to be safe and medically effective. Nearly two-thirds of the sample agreed with, or were neutral toward withholding coverage for medically effective high-cost technologies or treatments when less expensive and equally effective ones were available. The trade-offs the public would be willing to make on the basis of cost and effectiveness when considered together were not explored.[60]

More recently, President Obama's transition team invited the American public to meet in town halls to discuss pressing healthcare problems. Over 30 000 people participated in 3300 groups across the country. Although cost concerns figured prominently in issues identified by Americans, the discussion format was not designed to support in-depth considerations of approaches to problem solving. A section of the report that reported on solutions, however, describes the views of members of groups in California and New Mexico who believed that limiting coverage of expensive procedures with limited benefits was a way forward toward higher-value care. Many in attendance at the town hall meetings wished to remain engaged in healthcare reform and requested more opportunities to discuss the issues and consider background information and solutions.[61]

ROLES FOR THE PUBLIC: WHAT QUESTIONS SHOULD THEY TAKE ON?

In a recent interview with Barack Obama, the President reflected on the experience of his grandmother's death in the context of the issues it raised in making the US healthcare system accessible to all Americans. Terminally ill with cancer, Obama's grandmother fell last year and broke her hip. She died two weeks after undergoing hip-replacement surgery. Obama was quoted in a New York Times interview as saying: 'I don't know how much that hip replacement cost. I would have paid out of pocket for that hip replacement, just because she's my grandmother. Whether, sort of in the aggregate, society making those decisions to give my grandmother, or everybody else's ageing grandparents or parents, a hip replacement when they're terminally ill, is a sustainable model is a very difficult question.'[62]

Jonathan Lomas described the different perspectives members of the public can bring to discussions about healthcare priority setting when assuming the roles of: 'patient,' 'tax-payer,' and, 'collective decision maker.'[63] A patient comes with a very particular sense of investment in their available options in the context of illness. A taxpayer is concerned with the economic ramifications of decision making. The collective decision maker contributes their view of the actions that he or she believes would best serve the general good of the community. Collective decision makers are asked to examine their views from behind a 'veil of ignorance' in which they have no knowledge of what their future health needs are, and are thereby less likely to be motivated by self-interest.[18]

In the discussion of his grandmother's care, Obama reflected the implicit conflict inherent in these positions and the need to broaden participation in deliberations about a reformed healthcare system. He said: 'There is going to be a very difficult democratic conversation that takes place. It is very difficult to imagine the country making decisions just through normal political channels.'

Some political scientists have argued that policy is best made by those with technical expertise and that the electoral process provides sufficient opportunity for public input.[64,65] Specific to citizen participation in healthcare policy, questions have been raised about what participants can be effective at doing.[66,67] Others endorse public participation and public deliberation on policy issues as being democratising (i.e. non-elitist and leading to enhanced social solidarity), activating of citizenship and leading to better quality decisions.[68–70]

Judgements on clinical effectiveness and on healthcare financing and management are subjects on which technical expertise is integral to sound decision making. On the other hand, at its heart, setting priorities for limited healthcare resources is value based. And it is here at the fundamental level of 'what is fair?' that public representatives can provide guidance in setting coverage priorities.

In the case of CEA, it is well established that the use of cost-effectiveness ratios to determine coverage policy will be at variance with public values around distributive justice and equity.[57,71] This is because a simple cost-effectiveness ratio treats QALYs equally and trade-offs are not delineated between old and young, between better- and worse-off (economically and in terms of health status), and between improving quality of life and saving lives. The ethical and normative assumptions that are embedded in the ratios need to be examined more fully by the society for whom the resources are intended. If CEA is to become an acceptable input into coverage policy, citizens' views on value-based issues that accompany its use in priority setting become central.

A MODEL FROM ABROAD

Countries that have used CEA to inform coverage policy have studied public value structures and have implemented processes for bringing these views forward to decision makers.[72-77] NICE's 30-member Citizens Council serves as a means for incorporating the views of members of the public into its appraisal process.[78,79] Council members, who serve three-year terms, are recruited from a broad spectrum of the English and Welsh population. The Council meets semi-annually for a three-day period and deliberate on values that underpin NICE appraisal committee decisions. The Citizens Council has discussed issues including: whether age should enter into priority-setting considerations; how cost effectiveness should be taken into account in the case of premium prices for ultra-orphan drugs to treat rare diseases; trade-offs between saving the life of people in imminent danger of death versus improving the quality of life for others, or preventing disease later on. It has also been consulted on whether NICE guidance should be directed toward decreasing the gap in health status and longevity occasioned by socioeconomic status.

Predictably, examining the priorities of a cross-section of the public has not always yielded neat consensus statements by the Council's membership. People of differing faith, culture, socioeconomic status, and world view see things differently. But empirical work has shown that posing high-stakes questions to a diverse group that holds public accountability for the outcome of their decisions, motivates effective deliberative processes on the part of citizens.[80]

The Citizens Council is a conduit by which NICE's appraisal committees and leadership receive well-considered social value judgements from a cross-section of users of the NHS. NICE's Chairman, Sir Michael Rawlins, acknowledges that there will be instances when expert committee recommendations diverge from the views brought forward by the Citizens Council. However, the expectation is explicit that NICE's advisory groups will be guided by principles generated by the Council, and asked to provide justification for decisions that run contrary.[81]

HOW DO WE GATHER PUBLIC VIEWS ON HEALTHCARE PRIORITIES?

Capturing citizen views on healthcare priorities carries significant challenges. Earlier US efforts at public involvement at national and at state levels were criticised for relying on participant self-selection and the resulting homogeneity of occupation, education and race that frequently accompanies this method of outreach.[64,80,81] Similar concerns have been raised about the representativeness of the attendees at community meetings associated with the Oregon experiment.[65] An additional difficulty identified in previous attempts at meaningful engagement of the public was that consumers rarely received sufficient training or staff support to participate effectively in discussions with health professionals. Further, these discussions were typically directed at technical concerns, and values and normative issues on which the public can be said to be expert were rarely addressed explicitly.[82]

NICE's method for recruiting its Citizens Council relied on a community-based organisation that employed a broad outreach strategy. Members were selected to be as reflective as possible of the population of England and Wales.[68] This approach may hold lessons for the construction of such a group or groups advisory to US insurers.

Once advisory groups are formed, information must be provided to participants that allows them to examine and comfortably engage the issues they are presented with. Group members can be expected to lack experience with the practice of deliberation and resolution of issues within groups. These challenges require that public input be captured in a setting where neutral and comprehensible information is provided to participants. The process must also be facilitated by thoughtful independent parties. The political science literature and international work with citizen juries in health provides information on how to direct the process.[83,84]

The US healthcare system has been slow to involve Americans in a process that explores the allocation of healthcare spending in an equitable and affordable manner. The historical dominance of private insurance has delayed confrontation of the tension between universal coverage and affordability.

In the coming days of US healthcare reform, the Medicare programme, a programme that benefits all taxpayers, offers a logical meeting ground from which to engage the public in discussions that address fundamental values of 'who' and 'what' should gain priorities for coverage. The question of 'who' must factor in people's capacity to benefit from care; their level of suffering or disadvantage; their behavioural choices; and their age. 'What', must consider questions such as whether interventions that improve quality of life can be thought about in the same language (i.e. QALYs) as those that are life saving; whether we should prioritise investments in prevention or cure; and how effective a treatment must be in order to warrant coverage.

A logical place to convene these discussions is as council to the Medicare Evidence Development Coverage Advisory Committee (MedCAC).[85,86] The MedCAC does not consider cost-effectiveness information in making its recommendations, but it shares similar functions to those of NICE appraisal committees as advisers to national health programs. NICE's Citizens Council may provide a model for recruiting and structuring discussions with the public. The role of the Citizens Council has been to examine value-laden questions that follow from key issues on which CEA is silent; use of CEA has been a given from the start. Depending on the political environment, a US-constituted group might take the issue head-on, of whether CEA is an acceptable input to coverage decision making, thereby bringing this debate forward from the grassroots level. If the US reform process moves to incorporate CEA into coverage criteria (through CMS rule making, or congressional statute) public councillors could be asked to consider the contextual issues that should guide the use of CEA. Either way, media coverage of these discussions promises to foster a deeper understanding on the part of the public of what the choices are for Medicare. As they have done in England, these conversations can provoke a broader national dialogue on how to shape a more equitable and efficient healthcare system.

A review of the literature that has examined the attitudes of the public toward limit setting suggests that Americans understand and are prepared to engage in the issues that arise when setting priorities and imposing limits for their public programmes. This is in contrast to the perceptions of the policy community, and certainly to many in the for-profit medical industry that have most to gain materially from the current coverage approach that excludes examination of value received for money spent.[87]

Seemingly controversial approaches that are publicly vetted can give legislators more confidence in making needed changes. At a time when the political process has made so little progress in reforming the healthcare system, strategies for engaging the public and capturing its values, as NICE has developed, merit active pursuit in the US. These efforts will assist in crafting solutions to sustaining an equitable and efficient Medicare program, and more broadly, a healthcare system that provides for all Americans.

Acknowledgements

This chapter draws from work published earlier in: Gold MR, Sofaer S, Siegelberg T. Medicare and cost-effectiveness analysis: time to ask the taxpayers. *Health Aff (Millwood)*. 2007; **26**(5): 1399–406.

REFERENCES

1 OECD. *OECD Health Data 2009*. Paris: Organisation for Economic Cooperation and Development; 2009. Available at: www.oecd.org/dataoecd/46/2/38980580.pdf (accessed 22 September 2009).

2 Kaiser Family Foundation. *Health Coverage and the Uninsured: trends in health coverage*. Available at: www.kff.org/uninsured/trends.cfm (accessed 22 September 2009).

3 Hussey PS, Anderson GF, Osborn R, et al. How does the quality of care compare in five countries? *Health Aff (Millwood)*. 2004; **23**(3): 89–99.

4 Banks J, Marmot M, Oldfield Z, et al. Disease and disadvantage in the United States and in England. *JAMA*. 2006; **295**(17): 2037–45.

5 Nolte E, McKee CM. Measuring the health of nations: updating an earlier analysis. *Health Aff (Millwood)*. 2008; **27**(1): 58–71.

6 Congressional Budget Office. *The Long-Term Outlook for Healthcare Spending*. Washington: Congressional Budget Office; 2007. Available at: www.cbo.gov/ftpdocs/87xx/doc8758/mainText.3.1.shtml (accessed 22 September 2009).

7 Social Security and Medicare Boards of Trustees. *Summary of the 2006 Annual Reports*. Available at: www.socialsecurity.gov/OACT/TRSUM/index.html (accessed 21 August 2009).

8 American Association of Retired Persons Public Policy Institute. *Out-of-Pocket Spending on Healthcare by Medicare Beneficiaries Age 65 and Older in 2003.* Available at: http://assets.aarp.org/rgcenter/health/dd101_spending.pdf (accessed 22 September 2009).

9 Joyce B, Lau D. Medicare part D prescription drug benefit: an update. *Beuhler Center on Aging, Health & Society Newsletter.* 2009; **22**(1).

10 Gellad WF, Huskamp HA, Phillips KA, *et al.* How the new Medicare drug benefit could affect vulnerable populations. *Health Aff (Millwood).* 2006; **25**(1): 248–55.

11 Wennberg JE, Freeman JL, Culp WJ. Are hospital services rationed in New Haven or over-utilised in Boston? *Lancet.* 1987; **1**(8543): 1185–9.

12 Welch WP, Miller ME, Welch HG. Geographic variation in expenditures for physicians' services in the United States. *N Engl J Med.* 1993; **328**(9): 621–7.

13 Fisher ES, Wennberg DE, Stukel TA, *et al.* The implications of regional variations in Medicare spending. Part 1: the content, quality, and accessibility of care. *Ann Intern Med.* 2003; **138**(4): 273–87.

14 Fisher ES, Wennberg DE, Stukel TA, *et al.* The implications of regional variations in Medicare spending. Part 2: health outcomes and satisfaction with care. *Ann Intern Med.* 2003; **138**(4): 288–98.

15 Pear R. *US to compare medical treatments.* The New York Times; 16 February 2009.

16 Gottlieb S. *Congress Wants to Restrict Drug Access: a bill in the house could tie your doctor's hands.* Wall Street Journal; 20 January 2009.

17 Avorn J. Debate about funding comparative-effectiveness research. *N Engl J Med.* 2009; **360**(19): 1927–9.

18 Russell LB, Gold MR, Siegel JE, *et al.* The role of cost-effectiveness analysis in health and medicine: panel on cost-effectiveness in health and medicine. *JAMA.* 1996; **276**(14): 1172–7.

19 Neumann PJ. *Using Cost-Effectiveness Analysis to Improve Healthcare.* New York, NY: Oxford University Press; 2005.

20 Siegel JE. Cost-effectiveness analysis in US healthcare decision making: where is it going? *Med Care.* 2005; **43**(7 Suppl.): 1–4.

21 Henry DA, Hill SR, Harris A. Drug prices and value for money: the Australian Pharmaceutical Benefits Scheme. *JAMA.* 2005; **294**(20): 2630–2.

22 Oberlander J, Marmor T, Jacobs L. Rationing medical care: rhetoric and reality in the Oregon Health Plan. *CMAJ.* 2001; **164**(11): 1583–7.

23 Pearson SD, Rawlins MD. Quality, innovation, and value for money: NICE and the British National Health Service. *JAMA.* 2005; **294**(20): 2618–22.

24 Whalen J. *Valued Lives: Britain stirs outcry by weighing benefits of drugs versus price.* Wall Street Journal; 22 November 2005.

25 Personal communication: Michael D Rawlins, Chairman NICE; 12 March 2006.

26 Neumann PJ, Rosen AB, Weinstein MC. Medicare and cost-effectiveness analysis. *N Engl J Med.* 2005; **353**(14): 1516–22.

27 Gillick MR. Medicare coverage for technological innovations: time for new criteria? *N Engl J Med.* 2004; **350**(21): 2199–203.

28 Foote SB. Why Medicare cannot promulgate a national coverage rule: a case of regula mortis. *J Health Polit Policy Law.* 2002; **27**(5): 707–30.

29 Drummond MF, Jefferson TO. Guidelines for authors and peer reviewers of economic sub-missions to the BMJ: the BMJ Economic Evaluation Working Party. *BMJ.* 1996; **313**(7052): 275–83.

30 Garber AM. Cost-effectiveness and evidence evaluation as criteria for coverage policy. *Health Aff (Millwood).* 2004; Suppl Web Exclusives: W4–284–96.

31 Gold MR, Siegel JE, Russell LB, *et al. Cost-Effectiveness in Health and Medicine.* New York, NY: Oxford University Press; 1996.

32 Weinstein MC, Siegel JE, Gold MR, *et al.* Recommendations of the panel on cost-effectiveness in health and medicine. *JAMA.* 1996; **276**(15): 1253–8.

33 Kassirer JP, Angell M. The journal's policy on cost-effectiveness analyses. *N Engl J Med.* 1994; **331**(10): 669–70.

34 Tunis SR. Why Medicare has not established criteria for coverage decisions. *N Engl J Med.* 2004; **350**(21): 2196–8.

35 Astrue MJ. Pseudoscience and the law: the case of the Oregon Medicaid rationing experiment. *Issues Law Med.* 1994; **9**(4): 375–86.

36 Eddy DM. Clinical decision making: from theory to practice. Applying cost-effectiveness analysis. The inside story. *JAMA.* 1992; **268**(18): 2575–82.

37 Garber AM. Evidence-based coverage policy. *Health Aff (Millwood).* 2001; **20**(5): 62–82.

38 Al MJ, Feenstra T, Brouwer WB. Decision makers' views on healthcare objectives and budget constraints: results from a pilot study. *Health Policy.* 2004; **70**(1): 33–48.

39 Aspinall SL, Good B, Glassman PA, *et al.* The evolving use of cost-effectiveness analysis in formulary management within the Department of Veteran's Affairs. *Med Care.* 2005; **43**(7 Suppl.): 20–6.

40 Luce BR. What will it take to make cost-effectiveness analysis acceptable in the United States? *Med Care.* 2005; **43**(7 Suppl.): 44–8.

41 Saha S, Hoerger TJ, Pignone MP, *et al.* The art and science of incorporating cost effectiveness into evidence-based recommendations for clinical preventive services. *Am J Prev Med.* 2001; **20**(3 Suppl.): 36–43.

42 WellPoint. *WellPoint National Pharmacy & Therapeutics Committee (P&T Committee).* Available at: www.wellpointnextrx.com/shared/noapplication/f1/s0/t0/pw_ad080629.pdf (accessed 22 September 2009).

43 Aaron HJ, Schwartz WB. *Can We Say No? the challenge of rationing healthcare.* Washington, DC: Brookings Institution Press; 2005.

44 Russel S. *Oregon Stirs Controversy.* San Francisco, CA: San Francisco Chronicle; 27 April 1992.

45 McCall W. *Cystic Fibrosis Teen Faces Tough Odds, No Matter How They're Added Up.* Associated Press; 8 June 2000.

46 Leichter HM. Oregon's bold experiment: whatever happened to rationing? *J Health Polit Policy Law.* 1999; **24**(1): 147–60.

47 Goold SD, Green SA, Biddle AK, *et al.* Will insured citizens give up benefit coverage to include the uninsured? *J Gen Intern Med.* 2004; **19**(8): 868–74.

48 Danis M, Biddle AK, Goold SD. Insurance benefit preferences of the low-income uninsured. *J Gen Intern Med.* 2002; **17**(2): 125–33.

49 Danis M, Biddle AK, Goold SD. Enrollees choose priorities for Medicare. *Gerontologist* 2004; **44**(1): 58–67.

50 Personal communication: Susan Dorr Goold; 3 August 2008.

51 Sacramento Healthcare Decisions. *Cost-Effectiveness as a Criterion for Medical and Coverage Decisions: understanding and responding to community perspectives.* Sacramento, CA: Sacramento Healthcare Decisions; 2004. Available at: http://chcd.org/docs/vf.pdf (accessed 26 October 2009)

52 Ginsburg ME. Cost-effectiveness: will the public buy it or balk? *Health Aff (Millwood).* 2004; (Suppl. Web Exclusives): W4–297.

53 Sacramento Healthcare Decisions. *Getting Good Value: Consumers Debate Costly Treatments: is the gain worth the expense.* Sacramento, CA: Sacramento Healthcare Decisions; 2006. Available at: www.chcd.org/docs/ggv_report.pdf (accessed 26 October 2009)

54 Gold M, Franks P, Siegelberg T, *et al.* Does providing cost-effectiveness information change coverage priorities for citizens acting as social decision makers? *Health Policy.* 2006; **83**(1): 65–72.

55 Williams A. Intergenerational equity: an exploration of the 'fair innings' argument. *Health Econ.* 1997; **6**(2): 117–32.

56 Hadorn DC. Setting healthcare priorities in Oregon: cost-effectiveness meets the rule of rescue. *JAMA.* 1991; **265**(17): 2218–25.

57 Menzel P, Gold MR, Nord E, *et al.* Toward a broader view of values in cost-effectiveness analysis of health. *Hastings Cent Rep.* 1999; **29**(3): 7–15.
58 Cookson R, Dolan P. Public views on healthcare rationing: a group discussion study. *Health Policy.* 1999; **49**(1–2)6: 3–74.
59 Bryan S, Sofaer S, Siegelberg T, *et al.* Has the time come for cost-effectiveness analysis in US healthcare? Health Econ Policy Law. 2009; **4**(4): 425–43. Epub 2009 February 9.
60 Citizens' Healthcare Working Group. *Citizens' Healthcare Working Group Interim Recommendations.* Available at: http://govinfo.library.unt.edu/chc/recommendations/execsumm.html (accessed 22 September 2009).
61 US Department of Health and Human Services. *Americans Speak on Health Reform: Report on Healthcare Community Discussions.* 2009. Available at: www.healthreform.gov/reports/hccd/report_on_communitydiscussions.pdf (accessed 24 September 2009).
62 Baker P. *Personal Experience Weighs on Obama in Health Policy Debate.* The New York Times; 1 May 2009.
63 Lomas J. Reluctant rationers: public input to healthcare priorities. *J Health Serv Res Policy.* 1997; **2**(2): 103–11.
64 Nagel JH. Combining deliberation and fair representation in community health decisions. *Univ PA Law Rev.* 1992; **140**(5): 1965–85.
65 Schumpter J. *Capitalism, Socialism and Democracy.* 3rd ed. New York, NY: Harper Collins; 1984.
66 Rifkin SB. Lessons from community participation in health programmes. *Health Policy Plan.* 1986; **1**(3): 240–9.
67 Church J, Saunders D, Wanke M, *et al.* Citizen participation in health decision-making: past experience and future prospects. *J Public Health Policy.* 2002; **23**(1): 12–32.
68 Davies C, Wetherell M, Barnett E, *et al. Opening the Box: evaluating the Citizens' Council of NICE. Report prepared for the National Coordinating Centre for Research Methodology, NHS Research and Development Programme.* Milton Keynes: The Open University; March 2005.
69 Barber B. *Strong Democracy: participatory politics for a new age.* Berkeley, CA: University of California Press; 1984.
70 Gutman A, Thompson D. *Why Deliberative Democracy.* Princeton, NJ: Princeton University Press; 2004.
71 Daniels N. Equity and population health: toward a broader bioethics agenda. *Hastings Cent Rep.* 2006; **36**(4): 22–35.
72 Bowie C, Richardson A, Sykes W. Consulting the public about health service priorities. *BMJ.* 1995; **311**(7013): 1155–8.
73 Abelson J, Forest PG, Eyles J, *et al.* Deliberations about deliberative methods: issues in the design and evaluation of public participation processes. *Soc Sci Med.* 2003; **57**(2): 239–51.
74 Dolan P, Cookson R, Ferguson B. Effect of discussion and deliberation on the public's views of priority setting in healthcare: focus group study. *BMJ.* 1999; **318**(7188): 916–19.
75 Bowling A, Jacobson B, Southgate L. Explorations in consultation of the public and health professionals on priority setting in an inner London health district. *Soc Sci Med.* 1993; **37**(7): 851–7.
76 Bryan S, Roberts T, Heginbotham C, *et al.* QALY-maximisation and public preferences: results from a general population survey. *Health Econ.* 2002; **11**(8): 679–93.
77 Gold MR. Tea, biscuits, and healthcare prioritising. *Health Aff (Millwood).* 2005; **24**(1): 234–9.
78 National Institute for Health and Clinical Excellence. *Social Value Judgements: principles for the development of NICE guidance.* London: NIHCE; 2005. Available at: www.nice.org.uk/media/873/2F/SocialValueJudgementsDec05.pdf (accessed 22 September 2009).
79 Rawlins MD. Pharmacopolitics and deliberative democracy. *Clin Med.* 2005; **5**(5): 471–5.

80 Ryfe DM. Does deliberative democracy work? *Annu Rev Polit Sci.* 2005; **8**: 49–71.

81 Morone J, Marmor T. Representing Consumer Interests: the case of American health planning. In: Checkoway B, editor. *Citizens and Health Care: participation and planning for social change.* New York, NY: Pergamon Press; 1981.

82 Sofaer S. Community health planning in the United States: a post-mortem. *Fam Community Health.* 1988; **10**(4): 1–12.

83 Delap C. *Making better decisions: report of an IPPR symposium, Citizen's Juries and other methods of public involvement.* London: Institute For Public Policy Research; 1998. p. 27.

84 Lenaghan J. Involving the public in rationing decisions: the experience of citizens' juries. *Health Policy.* 1999; **49**(1–2): 45–61.

85 Foote SB. Why Medicare cannot promulgate a national coverage rule: a case of regula mortis. *J Health Polit Policy Law.* 2002; **27**(5): 707–30.

86 Foote SB, Wholey D, Rockwood T, *et al.* Resolving the tug-of-war between Medicare's national and local coverage. *Health Aff (Millwood).* 2004; **23**(4): 108–23.

87 Fleck LM. The costs of caring: Who pays? Who profits? Who panders? *Hastings Cent Rep.* 2006; **36**(3): 13–17.

CHAPTER 17

Harvesting and publishing patients' unanswered questions about the effects of treatments

Mark Fenton, Anne Brice and Iain Chalmers

The beginning of wisdom is found in doubting; by doubting we come to the question, and by seeking we may come upon the truth.

Pierre Abélard (1079–1142)

BACKGROUND

Pierre Abélard observed a millennium ago that sceptical acknowledgement of uncertainty offers an important route to increase knowledge. Recognising uncertainty is particularly important in an applied field like healthcare because health professionals and policy makers have a history of doing more harm than good – sometimes on a massive scale – with interventions used with the best of intentions.[1]

Some uncertainties about the effects of treatments will always remain difficult or impossible to resolve. For example, however much information about the beneficial effects of a treatment may be available from past experience, it is usually impossible to predict with complete confidence whether individual patients will benefit.

Other kinds of uncertainty can be reduced by eliciting patients' preferences about treatment modes or outcomes. Patients who are terrified by the prospect of surgery under general anaesthesia, for example, may well prefer to opt for non-surgical treatments, even if the latter are less likely to reduce their health problems.

165

Health professionals and patients are sometimes uncertain about the effects of treatments because they are not aware of research that could resolve their uncertainties. As a consequence, some treatments have been used long after research has shown that they do more harm than good, while other treatments have been withheld for years after strong evidence has become available that they are life saving.[1,2] Although there has recently been an improvement in access to systematic reviews of research evidence, and guidelines based on them, there is still a long way to go before these 'unknown knowns' become 'known knowns' to all of those recommending or using interventions within health services.[3,4]

Finally, uncertainties about the effect of treatments often persist after all the relevant research evidence has been reviewed systematically – thus exposing 'known unknowns'. Patients have suffered because of the failure to acknowledge and address some of these uncertainties and the General Medical Council has recently made clear that doctors 'must help to resolve uncertainties about the effects of treatments'.[5,6]

Acknowledging 'known unknowns' about the effects of treatments

In 2003, the James Lind Initiative was established with support from the Medical Research Council (MRC) and the National Institute for Health Research (NIHR) to promote public and professional knowledge and discussion about, and involvement in, clinical trials.[7] Rather than attempt to address this challenge directly, however, a decision was taken to address it indirectly by drawing attention to the importance of acknowledging and addressing uncertainties about the effects of treatments.[8-11]

This emphasis has subsequently been adopted elsewhere. For example, the *BMJ* has launched a new series of articles drawing attention to uncertainties[12], and the NIHR Health Technology Assessment Programme had four subsections entitled 'Reducing Uncertainty' in its 2008 annual report.[13] The NIHR has also invested substantial funding in several Collaborations for Leadership in Applied Health Research and Care (CLAHRC), and these are beginning their work by soliciting unanswered questions for consideration as possible research priorities.

Involving patients and the public in prioritising research on the effects of treatments

As systematic reviews of research gradually cover the vast scope of clinical practice, they reveal just how many of the questions deemed important by clinicians and patients cannot be answered by the available research. The extent of the mismatch between the questions researchers have addressed and those that patients and clinicians would like answers to is unknown, but a survey of published reports by Sandy Oliver and Jennifer Gray leaves little room for complacency. They identified 334 studies documenting patients' or clinicians' priorities for research, but these priorities matched those of researchers in only six and three studies, respectively.[14]

An unsettling picture emerges from this effort to assess the extent to which researchers are meeting the information needs of those whose interests they often purport to serve. For example, researchers in Bristol investigated the extent to which research on the management of osteoarthritis of the knee was addressing questions deemed important by patients, and by the clinicians looking after them.[15] They convened four focus groups – of patients, rheumatologists, physiotherapists and GPs. All contributors made it clear that they had had enough of trials sponsored by pharmaceutical companies to compare yet more unneeded non-steroidal anti-inflammatory drugs against placebos. Yet these studies continue to dominate therapeutic research activity in this field. Instead of drug trials, patients and their carers wanted more rigorous evaluation of physiotherapy and surgery, and assessment of the educational and coping strategies that might help patients to manage this chronic, disabling and often painful condition more successfully.

Even when questions of importance to patients have been addressed, the outcomes that have been measured have not necessarily been those that patients would regard as most relevant. More than a decade ago, rheumatologists established an international group – Outcome Measures in Rheumatology Arthritis Clinical Trials (OMERACT) to reach agreement on a standard core of outcome measures in rheumatoid arthritis clinical trials. A few years ago they decided to invite patients to contribute to the group's discussions. A survey of patients revealed that pain was not the dominant symptom that concerned patients, as researchers had assumed. Fatigue was the symptom that topped the list, and this had been almost completely ignored by earlier researchers.[16]

The gap between perceived research priorities and unanswered questions that are deemed important to patients can be illustrated with a recommendation for further research in a NICE technology appraisal. The topic was inhaler devices for the routine treatment of chronic asthma in older children.[17] The only recommendation for research in this appraisal was the need to compare the relative merits of holding chambers versus nebulisers for inhaled drugs. By contrast, when the James Lind Alliance invited patients and parents of children to identify the most important uncertainties about treatments for asthma, their answers were dominated by concerns about the possible long-term adverse effects of chronic medication for asthma. Until recently,[18] there was no readily available synthesis of existing, reliable information. This uncertainty was not reflected in any of the readily accessible lists of research recommendations.

It is clear that researchers could do more to address patients' and clinicians' questions. What remains unclear is how, in a research world where perverse incentives often determine what research will be done,[19] the information needs of patients and clinicians can achieve more prominence.[20]

THE UK DATABASE OF UNCERTAINTIES ABOUT THE EFFECTS OF TREATMENTS

Rationale and inclusion criteria

Numerous questions about the effects of treatments have not yet been investigated in systematic reviews of existing evidence, and numerous systematic reviews have shown that the evidence fails to resolve many important questions. The UK Database of Uncertainties about the Effects of Treatments (UK DUETs) was created to publish these 'known unknowns' about the effects of treatments, and to draw attention to any ongoing research designed to address them. UK DUETs thus provides a resource to help research funders such as the Health Technology Assessment Programme of the NIHR[13] and the MRC to prioritise uncertainties for new research – either in the form of new, extended or updated systematic reviews; or as additional 'primary' research.

For the purposes of UK DUETs, 'treatment uncertainties' are defined as 'uncertainties that cannot currently be answered by referring to reliable, up-to-date systematic reviews of existing research evidence'. Eligible uncertainties – 'known unknowns' – thus meet at least one of the following criteria, with implications for action noted in italics.

➤ No relevant systematic reviews identified – *implication: prepare systematic review(s).*
➤ Relevant reliable up-to-date systematic reviews do not address continuing uncertainties about treatment effects – *implication: extend existing systematic review(s).*
➤ Existing relevant systematic reviews are not up to date – *implication: update existing systematic review(s).*
➤ Reliable, up-to-date systematic reviews have revealed important continuing uncertainties about treatment effects – *implication: conduct additional primary research.*

Harvesting uncertainties

Despite a growing acceptance that it is important to be explicit about uncertainties regarding the effects of treatments, reluctance to do so remains widespread. For example, some of the people responsible for developing clinical guidelines do not consider it part of their brief to make uncertainties explicit or to propose further research to address them. By contrast, NICE has developed a research recommendations database of treatment uncertainties that have emerged during the process of developing a guideline.[21] The Cochrane Collaboration now provides guidance to those preparing systematic reviews on how to make uncertainties explicit, and recommendations for further research, in its *Reviewers' Handbook*.[22]

Uncertainties for inclusion in UK DUETs are sought in several sources, some of which yield their fruits more readily than others. Research recommendations in systematic reviews and clinical guidelines are becoming more readily accessible, though historically, they are often poorly structured. Information about ongoing research is slowly becoming more accessible as the registers of clinical trials improve their coverage.[23] By contrast, obtaining information about the uncertainties that matter to patients, carers and clinicians is far more challenging.

Uncertainties identified through patients' and carers' questions about treatment effects

At the time of writing, most of the treatment uncertainties identified from patients' and carers' questions published in UK DUETs relate to asthma, schizophrenia and urinary incontinence. Uncertainties have been identified in all of these fields using funded surveys, targeting respondents through patient and carer groups.

Asthma UK posted a survey to 120 'Speak up for Asthma' volunteers, to 225 parents and children who had attended 'Kick Asthma' breaks and to a random sample of 801 other patients and carers. The survey was also placed on the Asthma UK website for three months, and news feeds and targeted articles were used to solicit responses.

The Mental Health Research Network Wales (Rhwydwaith Ymchwil Lechyd Meddwl Cymru) sought uncertainties about the effects of treatments by sending email questionnaires to MIND Cymru and Hafal (the leading charity in Wales for people with severe mental illness and their carers, covering all 22 local health board areas), and distributed copies of their survey at conferences. The Research Network also advertised a web-based survey through email alerts and professional contacts, and links from the home pages of several relevant groups, including Rethink – a UK national mental health membership charity for people with serious mental illness.

Uncertainties about the effects of treatments for urinary incontinence were sought by the Bladder and Bowel Foundation, a UK charity. It posted a survey to 1000 members and also placed the survey on its website. The charity used its internet forum to encourage people to submit their questions and made the survey available through the websites of other relevant organisations. The Foundation also published web links in its own magazine, and those of other patient organisations, such as Cystitis and Overactive Bladder, and Coloplast.[24]

Survey questions often require interpretation, suggesting that an agreed terminology is needed for patients, health professionals and researchers to discuss uncertainties.

Questions implying uncertainties have to be checked to confirm that they do indeed reflect 'known unknowns'. Not infrequently, we have found that reliable answers to patients' questions already existed but had not been made available to them, thus emphasising the need to improve access to information about 'known knowns'.

Uncertainties identified through clinicians' questions about treatment effects

Sources of clinicians' uncertainties have been sought with varying success. We thought that clinical question and answer services would provide a rich source of uncertainties, and that every question that could not be answered by referring to an up-to-date reliable systematic review would be eligible for inclusion in UK DUETs. However, clinical question and answer services exist to provide information deemed likely to be helpful to the clinician, and this is not necessarily based on systematic reviews of reliable research evidence.

To obtain clinicians' uncertainties about asthma treatment, the UK DUETs editor worked with the British Thoracic Society. Together, they identified explicit statements that described the need for further research in clinical management guidelines, statements of continuing uncertainty from systematic reviews and in research recommendations. Sources used included the Scottish Intercollegiate Guidelines Network (SIGN), the British Thoracic Society guideline on the management of asthma, the Cochrane Library, the National Library for Health Primary Care Question Answering Service, and the ATTRACT Service.

To identify uncertainties about the effects of treatments for schizophrenia and other forms of mental illness, the Mental Health Research Network Wales collaborated with the UK Mental Health Research Network in a survey of health professionals in England and Wales, but this resulted in very few responses.

For urinary incontinence, surveys were done to identify recommendations for further research in treatment guidelines and systematic reviews. In addition, professional organisations were invited to submit uncertainties about the effects of treatments.

As with patients' and carers' questions about the effects of treatments, clinicians' questions need to be interpreted to identify what the treatment uncertainties actually are. And as with questions raised by patients and carers, some of the questions submitted by clinicians could be resolved by existing up-to-date systematic reviews, emphasising again the need to improve access to information about 'known knowns'.

Uncertainties revealed in systematic reviews and clinical guidelines

Systematic reviews, clinical guidelines (such as those published by SIGN and NICE), consensus documents and publications such as *BMJ Clinical Evidence* and *Clinical Knowledge Summaries* are fruitful sources of research recommendations, which, by implication, reflect uncertainties.

Some recommendations for research made by the authors of systematic reviews and clinical guidelines are quite specific about what is needed, but many are not.

Because of this widespread lack of specificity, we convened an advisory group representing these constituencies to agree how research recommendations could be improved. The consensus reached was that treatment uncertainties should be expressed in terms of six variables summarised in the acronym 'EPICOT' – existing Evidence, the type of Patient (or Population), the Intervention of interest, the relevant Comparator, the treatment Outcomes considered important, and the Timing of the judgement that the uncertainty existed. A detailed account of the advisory group's recommendations was published in the *BMJ* in 2006,[25] and there is encouraging evidence that it is being heeded.[26-30]

Uncertainties identified through information about ongoing research

Knowledge about uncertainties can be obtained from published information about ongoing research, either in the form of protocols for systematic reviews (such as those published in the *Cochrane Database of Systematic Reviews*), or in the clinical trials' registers accessible through the World Health Organization's International Clinical Trials Registry Platform – www.who.int/ictrp/en/

Guidance issued by the MRC and the Department of Health states that it is unethical as well as poor science to embark on new research without first finding out what is already known from existing evidence. Hence, new research should be commissioned only after it has been shown in reliable systematic reviews of existing research evidence that the additional research is needed and that it has been designed to take account of lessons from earlier research. Records of ongoing clinical trials that do not make reference to systematic reviews showing why the trial is justified are not included in UK DUETs.

Continuing challenges in identifying uncertainties

It must be clear from this account that methods to identify uncertainties about the effects of treatments remain relatively poorly explored. There is currently no justification to confidently promote any specific approach to collecting them. This particularly applies to methods for trying to identify uncertainties deemed important by patients, carers and clinicians. The strengths and limitations of the approaches that have been used thus far might be clarified by a more detailed analysis of the experiences described above and other studies seeking patients' and clinicians' priorities for research.[14] In light of experience so far, the James Lind Alliance is compiling a handbook to guide future priority-setting partnerships (PSPs) in the methods used to elicit uncertainties from patients, carers and clinicians.

Nevertheless, of the uncertainties contained in UK DUETs at the time of writing, 337 have been derived from patients' questions, 67 from carers' questions and 94 from clinicians' questions. Research recommendations were the source of 716 uncertainties, and 105 were made explicit in records of ongoing research.

Assembling, organising, publishing and downloading information about the uncertainties in UK DUETs

Each potential UK DUETs entry needs to be assessed to check if there are any up-to-date, reliable systematic reviews addressing the uncertainty (the Evidence of EPICOT). Judgements about reliability are made using the DC-QC INDEX, which has been piloted and published by cancer specialists working in the National Library for Health.[31] If no up-to-date, reliable, systematic reviews can be found, it implies that an uncertainty is eligible for inclusion in UK DUETs. If one or more relevant systematic reviews exist, they need to be checked to ensure that they are reliable and up to date, and if so, what the authors concluded. *See* Figure 17.1 for a schematic version of the process.

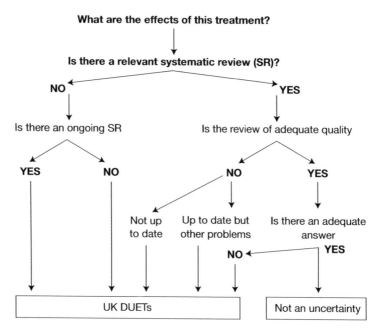

FIGURE 17.1: Decision tree to guide addition of uncertainties to UK DUETs.

The key elements of each treatment uncertainty entered in UK DUETs cover the remaining elements indicated by the EPICOT acronym. The title of the uncertainty often includes the Patient (or Population); it usually contains the intervention, often the Comparator, and sometimes the specific Outcomes of interest. The date the record was added provides the Timing of the judgement that the uncertainty existed.

When possible, the original text that expressed the uncertainty is included in the UK DUETs record so users can check if any meaning has been lost through editing. UK DUETs records also include citations for any systematic reviews that meet the inclusion criteria of being up to date, or in need of updating or extending, and links to ongoing research (whether systematic reviews or new studies) that appears to address the uncertainty.

Figure 17.2 provides an example of how a UK DUETs record is displayed. Further details of the information recorded can be seen on UK DUETs website: www.library.nhs.uk/DUETs. Records can be exported into spreadsheets.

NHS Evidence - UK Database of Uncertainties about the Effects of Treatments (DUETs)

NHS Evidence Home > Specialist Collections >
UK Database of Uncertainties about the Effects of Treatments (DUETs) Home

What is the best way of dealing with allergies to cats & dogs to prevent asthma?

Record type	Uncertainties identified from patients' questions
Source	Asthma UK Adviceline
Why is there uncertainty?	Reliable up-to-date systematic reviews have revealed important continuing uncertainties about treatment effects
References to reliable up-to-date systematic reviews:	Kilburn S, Lasserson TJ, McKean M. Pet allergen control measures for allergic asthma in children and adults. Cochrane Database of Systematic Reviews 2001, Issue 1. Art. No.: CD002989. DOI: 10.1002/14651858.CD002989.
What is needed?	Further research
Systematic reviews that need updating or extending	Abramson MJ, Puy RM, Weiner JM. Allergen immunotherapy for asthma. Cochrane Database of Systematic Reviews 2003, Issue 4. Art. No.: CD001186. DOI: 10.1002/14651858.CD001186.
Systematic reviews in preparation	*None identified*
Ongoing controlled trials	Manchester Asthma and Allergy Study - Primary prevention of asthma and allergy by allergen avoidance in high risk infants ISRCTN63558189
	Prevention of asthma in children at high risk of developing asthma ISRCTN ISRCTN66748327
	Air cleaners for children and adolescents with asthma and dog allergy NCT00220753

Classification

Which health conditions?	
What is person's age?	Any age
Which types of treatments?	Education and training Environmental
Which outcomes?	Minimal symptoms with minimal need for reliever medication; no exacerbations; no limitation on physical activity and normal lung function.

Record ID: 302741   **Publication date:** 03 Jul 2007

Last reviewed date: 03 Jul 2007   **Publication type:** Known Uncertainty

The DUETs team endeavours to ensure that information is correct at the time of data entry.

NHS Evidence – provided by NICE | Usage & Privacy
Policy | Feedback | Accessibility

FIGURE 17.2: UK DUETs record.

DEVELOPING AND MAINTAINING UK DUETS

An infrastructure was needed to roll out the UK DUETs pilot, so that it could be extended and maintained, as existing uncertainties became resolved and new uncertainties emerged. Figure 17.3 shows that the current coverage of UK DUETs is patchy. Information wealth (for example, in the UK DUETs asthma module) sits side by side with information poverty in most fields.

Cancer – All (46)
    Head and neck cancer (6)
    Lung cancer (4)
    Prostate cancer (1)
    Skin cancer (7)
    Colorectal cancer (7)
    Oesophageal cancer (0)
    Stomach cancer (3)
Cardiovascular disease – All (45)
    Heart disease (31)
      Myocardial ischaemia (2)
      Heart failure (17)
    Stroke (5)
Ear, nose and throat disorders – All (116)
    Hearing disorders (19)
    Otitis media (17)
    Rhinitis (18)
    Tonsillitis (8)
Eyes and vision – All (13)
    Age-related macular degeneration (11)
Gastroenterological and liver diseases – All (57)
Haematological disorders – All (7)
Infection – All (12)
Mental health – All (177)
    Depression (9)
    Learning disabilities (3)
    Schizophrenia (153)
Musculoskeletal diseases – All (41)
Neonatal diseases (11)
Neurological conditions – All (102)
    Epilepsy (87)

Nutritional metabolic & endocrine disorders – All (89)
    Diabetes (59)
    Thyroid disorders (11)
Oral and dental conditions – All (8)
Respiratory diseases – All (322)
    Asthma (316)
Skin disorders – All (118)
    Acne vulgaris (1)
    Atopic eczema (59)
    Psoriasis (1)
    Skin cancer (7)
    Skin infections (4)
    Vitiligo (29)
Symptoms – All (3)
Trauma – All (4)
Urological and genital disorders – All (147)
    Kidney diseases (16)
    Urinary incontinence (130)
      Enuresis (14)
      Mixed (2)
      Neurogenic (15)
      Nocturia (5)
      Overactive bladder (8)
      Retention (2)
      Stress (14)
      Urge (7)
Women's health conditions – All (85)
    Endometriosis (35)
    Pregnancy and childbirth (21)
      Hypertension in pregnancy (1)

FIGURE 17.3: UK DUETs coverage, August 2009 (numbers of records in parentheses).

It was agreed in late 2006 that the National Library for Health provided the most appropriate infrastructure within the UK for developing and maintaining UK DUETs modules. Now part of NHS Evidence, specialist teams are responsible for assessing the prevalence and incidence of evidence for their respective spheres of responsibility. As well as organising these specialist collections of evidence based on explicit quality standards and protocols, the specialist teams are supported by editorial and advisory groups that represent key stakeholders in their respective communities, including professional organisations and societies, policy leads and patient groups. These channels for engaging with clinicians and clinical networks, and with patient organisations, have provided an important infrastructure for raising awareness of, and harvesting uncertainties.

Because their engagement with users has highlighted gaps in the coverage of their core evidence sources, the specialist teams were already aware of the importance of unanswered questions and uncertainties, and they became an obvious channel for the development and maintenance of UK DUETs modules. As well as keeping their specialist collections up to date, each team is responsible for summarising evidence in annual evidence updates covering, between them, 60 key health problems. This means that they are well placed to harvest uncertainties as part of their existing workflow and processes, for instance by adapting their search protocols for annual evidence updates to create UK DUETs records as a by-product, and to incorporate these in UK DUETs modules. *See* Figure 17.4 for a schematic illustration of this process.

Against this background, the invitation to tender for National Library for Health specialist libraries specified that, from April 2008, all health-condition-based specialist libraries 'must identify and publish uncertainties about the effects of treatments, using agreed procedures, through the DUETs.' This requirement was reflected in contracts, which specify that the provider 'agrees to work with the central team and DUETs to devise an agreed plan for contributing to the maintenance and development of DUETs modules,' and that one of the deliverables is to be a 'DUETs module in development'. Not only do these modules serve as components of UK DUETs, but they also contribute to each specialist group's more-specific-evidence collections. These developments demonstrate a recognition that it is important to present information about what is *not* known in the context of what is known.

INTEGRATING INFORMATION ABOUT 'KNOWN UNKNOWNS' WITH INFORMATION ABOUT 'KNOWN KNOWNS' IN NHS EVIDENCE AND NHS CHOICES

Information about what is and is not known about the effects of treatments is clearly relevant both to patients and to clinicians considering choices and making decisions about treatment. Yet not all such decision makers consider using

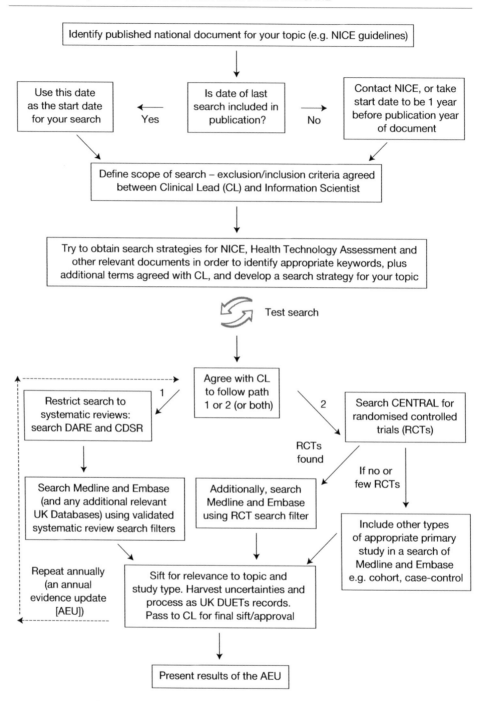

FIGURE 17.4: Annual evidence update flow chart.

evidence to be important or necessary, even when they know it exists. The NHS itself does not explicitly require it and the absence of a systematic approach to enabling it frustrates the development of a culture in which its use is easy and routine. A large number of enterprises, many funded and some operated by the NHS, generate, interpret and present evidence. Despite this, NHS decision makers often find it difficult to access what they need when they are at the point of making a decision. What they do access is not necessarily up to date and is of variable quality (both the original studies and the way in which they have been interpreted).

It is against this background that NHS Evidence and NHS Choices were created. Among other objectives, both these initiatives aim to improve access to evidence likely to be reliable for both clinicians and patients, and to foster shared decision making between them. In 2007, Lord Darzi, then a minister of health in the House of Lords, announced in an interim report:

'A national clinical evidence base will be created, housing what local, national and international clinicians believe to be the best available evidence about clinical practice, pathways and models of care and innovations. This will be available to commissioners, practitioners, patients and the public alike'.[32]

Following further consultation and a review of existing evidence services, Lord Darzi's final report declared:

'All NHS staff will have access to a new NHS Evidence service where they will be able to get, through a single web-based portal, authoritative clinical and non-clinical evidence and best practice'.[33]

NHS Evidence was created to provide a single gateway for all the professionals in the NHS who make decisions about treatments or the use of resources. It will also be openly available for patients who want to know more about their options for care. The model builds on the existing functions and capabilities of NICE and the National Library for Health, and their specialist groups. In addition to drawing much of its evidence base from the output of the research community, NHS Evidence will be able to identify gaps in knowledge and feed through suggestions for research topics. Figure 17.5 illustrates how known uncertainties feed into the overall quality framework for the organisation and presentation of sources. We are encouraged by the results of surveys of users and advisers to NHS Evidence Specialist Collections conducted in 2009. Building the content of UK DUETs was rated second only in importance to Annual Evidence Updates.

NHS Choices was developed to help patients and the public make informed choices about their health, from lifestyle decisions about things like smoking, drinking and exercise, through to the practical aspects of finding and using NHS services when they are needed. To ensure a supply of the best available evidence to inform treatment choices, the NHS Choices provider is required to use an explicit, consistent and systematic system for searching, sourcing and authoring

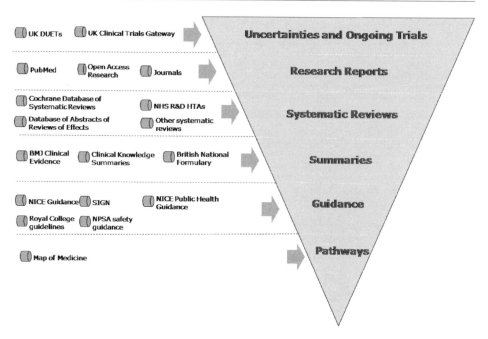

FIGURE 17.5: How known uncertainties feed into the overall quality framework for the organisation and presentation of sources (adapted from NHS Evidence commissioning papers).

content, based on the supply of knowledge provided by NHS Evidence. The process includes clear guidance for editors, authors and other providers of content, including searching protocols, compliance with indexing and metadata standards. Like NHS Evidence, NHS Choices encourages explicit acknowledgement of uncertainties and provides links to UK DUETs.

In addition to making uncertainties explicit, both NHS Evidence and NHS Choices will also provide information about ongoing research that addresses some of these uncertainties, and thus opportunities for patients and clinicians to contribute to these initiatives.[34] These developments offer exciting opportunities to help promote a culture in which research becomes embedded in the ethos and everyday practice of the NHS.

The challenge of meeting the information needs of clinicians and patients is far from complete, and patients continue to suffer unnecessarily as a result. This challenge will not go away – indeed, resolving one uncertainty almost always results in the recognition of additional uncertainties.[5] Nevertheless, we hope that, within a few years, professionals, patients and others will have ready access to reliable information on what is known about the effects of treatments, what is not known and what is being done to address important uncertainties.

Acknowledgements

We are grateful to Hazim Timimi for designing the database; members of UK DUETs Development Group (Jon Brassey, Polly Brown, Klara Brunnhuber, Kalipso Chalkidou, Mike Clarke, Julie Glanville, Paul Glasziou, Nick J Hicks, Mig Mueller, Ron Stamp, Mark Starr, David Tovey, Sara Twaddle, Chris Watkins and Pamela Young); the UK DUETs Pioneers (Ray Armstrong, Anne Brice, April Coombe, Douglas Grindlay, Angus Leitch, Nicola Pearce Smith, Steve Sharp); and to Angus Leitch, Gill Leng and Alison Turner for providing comments on earlier drafts of this chapter.

REFERENCES

1 Chalmers I. The lethal consequences of failing to make use of all relevant evidence about the effects of medical treatments: the need for systematic reviews. In: Rothwell P, editor. *Treating Individuals*. London: Lancet; 2007.

2 Antman EM, Lau J, Kupelnick B, *et al.* A comparison of results of meta-analyses of randomised control trials and recommendations of clinical experts: treatments for myocardial infarction. *JAMA.* 1992; **268**: 240–8.

3 Chalmers I, Glasziou P. Avoidable waste in the production and reporting of research evidence. *Lancet.* 2009; **374**(9683): 86–9.

4 Bastian H, Glasziou P, Chalmers I. Seventy-five trials and eleven systematic reviews a day: how will we ever cope? In press.

5 Chalmers I. Confronting therapeutic ignorance. *BMJ.* 2008; **337**: a841.

6 General Medical Council. *Good Medical Practice.* Available at: www.gmc-uk.org/guidance/good_medical_practice/index.asp (accessed 22 September 2009).

7 Chalmers I. The James Lind Initiative. *J R Soc Med.* 2003; **96**: 575–6.

8 Chalmers I. Well-informed uncertainties about the effects of treatments: how should clinicians and patients respond? *BMJ.* 2004; **328**: 475–6.

9 Chalmers I. Managers should help to address important uncertainties about the effects of treatments. *British Association of Medical Managers News.* 2004; June 3–4.

10 Lloyd K, Rose D, Fenton M. Identifying uncertainties about the effects of treatments for schizophrenia. *J Ment Health.* 2006; **15**(3): 263–8.

11 Chalmers I. Addressing uncertainties about the effects of treatments offered to NHS patients: whose responsibility? *J R Soc Med.* 2007; **100**(10): 440–1.

12 Chalmers I. How often do researchers address questions of interest to clinicians and patients? [letter from the editor] *BMJ Clin Evid.* 2008; 28 January.

13 NIHR HTA Programme. Developing research topics. In: *Update 2008. NIHR Coordinating Centre for Health Technology Assessment.* 2008; p. 4.

14 Oliver S, Gray J. *A Bibliography of Research Reports About Patients', Clinicians' and Researchers' Priorities for New Research.* Oxford: James Lind Alliance; 2006.

15 Tallon D, Chard J, Dieppe P. Relation between agendas of the research community and the research consumer. *Lancet.* 2000; **355**(9220): 2037–40.

16 Kirwan JR, Hewlett SE, Heiberg T, *et al.* Incorporating the patient perspective into outcome assessment in rheumatoid arthritis – progress at OMERACT 7. *J Rheumatol.* 2005; **32**: 2250–6.

17 National Institute for Health and Clinical Excellence. *Inhaler Devices for Routine Treatment of Chronic Asthma in Older Children (Aged 5–15 Years): NICE technology appraisal no. 38.* London: NIHCE; 2002.

18 Cates CJ, Cates MJ. Regular treatment with salmeterol for chronic asthma: serious adverse events. *Cochrane Database Syst Rev.* 2008; **3**: CD006363.

19 Chalmers I. Current controlled trials: an opportunity to help improve the quality of clinical research. *Curr Control Trials Cardiovasc Med.* 2000; **1**(1): 3–8.

20 Chalmers R, Jobling R, Chalmers I. Is the NHS willing to help clinicians and patients reduce uncertainties about the effects of treatments? *Clin Med.* 2005; **5**(3): 230–4.

21 National Institute for Health and Clinical Excellence. *NICE Guidance Research Recommendations.* London: NIHCE. Available at: www.nice.org.uk/research/index.jsp?action=rr (accessed 23 September 2009).

22 The Cochrane Collaboration. *Cochrane Handbook for Systematic Reviews of Interventions Version 5.0.1.* Higgins JPT, Green S, editors. Chichester, West Sussex; Hoboken, NJ: Wiley-Blackwell; 2008.

23 Ghersi D, Pang T. En route to international clinical trial transparency. *Lancet.* 2008; **372**(9649): 1531–2.

24 James Lind Initiative. *James Lind Alliance – Urinary Incontinence, Tackling treatment uncertainties together: report of the final priority setting workshop.* Oxford: James Lind Alliance; 2008.

25 Brown P, Brunnhuber K, Chalkidou K, *et al.* How to formulate research recommendations. *BMJ.* 2006; **333**(7572): 804–6.

26 Cook A. Subclinical hypothyroidism: let's identify research questions. *BMJ.* 2008; **337**: a1259.

27 Chalkidou K, Walley T, Culyer A, *et al.* Evidence-informed evidence-making. *J Health Serv Res Policy.* 2008; **13**: 167–73.

28 Holden G, Thyer BA, Baer J, *et al.* Suggestions to Improve Social Work Journal Editorial and Peer-Review Processes: the San Antonio response to the Miami statement. *Res Soc Work Pract.* 2008; **18**: 66–71.

29 Nicholson PJ. How to undertake a systematic review in an occupational setting. *Occup Environ Med.* 2007; **64**(5): 353–8.

30 Croft AM. A lesson learnt: the rise and fall of Lariam and Halfan. *J R Soc Med.* 2007; **100**(4): 170–4.

31 NHS Evidence. *Systematic Review Screening Tool.* Available at: http://stage.library.nhs.uk/Cancer/Page.aspx?pagename=DCQCINDEX (accessed 23 September 2009).

32 Darzi A. *NHS Next Stage Review Interim Report.* London: Department of Health; 2007.

33 Darzi A. *High Quality Care for All: NHS next stage review final report.* Cm. 7432. London: Department of Health; 2008.

34 Godlee F, Chalmers I. User-friendly, public information about all UK clinical trials: still not generally available. *BMJ.* 2009. In press.

CHAPTER 18

The future of patient and public involvement: some concluding thoughts

Peter Littlejohns, Marcia Kelson and Victoria Thomas

You have the right to be involved, directly or through representatives, in the planning of healthcare services, the development and consideration of proposals for changes in the way those services are provided and in decisions to be made affecting the operation of those services.

NHS constitution (21 January 2009)[1]

The NHS is accountable to the people, communities and patients that it serves. In this book we have tried to reflect a number of ways in which patients, carers and the public – both organisations and individuals – can contribute to the development of NICE guidance and its implementation support activities.

NICE consults with national patient, carer, community and voluntary organisations (including those that represent equality groups and public health issues) at all key stages of guidance development. All NICE advisory bodies include at least two lay members who have a remit to ensure that guidance takes into account patient and public issues, outcomes and preferences. NICE also ensures that patient views directly inform the discussions of its advisory bodies. For example, NICE invites patient experts to provide personal testimony at technology appraisal meetings and community experts to speak at public health advisory committee meetings. We also survey the views of patients by questionnaire for our interventional procedures guidance.

We have used a range of methods to collect information on patients' views when our advisory body has indicated that information is lacking in the published research literature. Examples include: focus groups with patients and service users in the development of clinical guidelines on heart failure, multiple sclerosis and self harm; workshops for young people with diabetes; and surveys at patient conferences for lung cancer and young people with cancer. Complementing all this is the role of our Citizens Council, which NICE uses as a sounding board to ensure that the views of the taxpayer are also obtained alongside organisations and individuals with a direct and vested interest in a specific guidance topic.

NICE is continually taking on responsibility for new activities. Recent examples include being invited by the Department of Health to produce Quality and Outcome Framework indicators and guidance on medical devices and quality standards. NICE has also been asked to work with the Department of Health to assess potential risk-sharing schemes developed by the pharmaceutical industry to make their products cost effective for use in the NHS. As we embark on these new activities, we will continue to ensure that opportunities for patient and public involvement are considered and, where relevant and workable, integrated into the process.

Patient and public involvement at NICE is just one facet of wider national and international attempts to engage more systematically with patients and the public. The need to involve patients and the public in UK health policy making and the planning and development of services is promoted by patient and carer organisations. It also features as a requirement in key NHS policy documents[2-5] and has recently been reinforced in the NHS Constitution.[1] Health inquiry reports have identified the (sometimes serious) limitations of neglecting to engage directly with those who are on the receiving end of policies, guidance and services in their development and implementation.[6,7]

There has been a renewed impetus following serious failings in emergency care provided by the Mid Staffordshire NHS Foundation Trust between 2005 and mid-2008. A review of this trust found that a significant reason that such poor care went unchecked for so long was that patients were not listened to. The review concluded that patients' views need to be a top priority in shaping and guiding the services provided in all NHS organisations. This should not just be the preserve of a small number of organisations exhibiting best practice, but should be systematic everywhere.[8] At NICE, we aim to ensure that patient and public views inform the development of NICE guidance so that it is evidence based and also patient centred. The guidance is issued to the NHS to underpin the provision of care and to shape services at a local level.

At an international level, healthcare systems are beset with the same problems facing the NHS, namely, ongoing developments and innovation in treatments, often expensive ones, within the context of finite healthcare budgets. As increasingly difficult decisions need to be taken, it becomes imperative to ensure that patient and public views inform policy decision making. Other healthcare systems are increasingly looking to NICE to identify ways in which difficult decisions about access to treatment can be taken that are robust, transparent, independent and inclusive. We hope that the chapters in this book provide an introduction to how patients and the public can contribute to this.

NICE materials and resources have always been publicly available on our website and on request. However, the number of requests for advice, information and materials from international bodies responsible for developing health policy has for some time exceeded the capacity of NICE staff to meet these demands. For this reason we recently set up an international consulting arm that can be commissioned to provide advice on how to develop clinically effective and cost-effective evidence-based guidance. This can include advice on developing and integrating approaches to patient and public involvement.

THE CITIZENS COUNCIL

When NICE was first established, one of its fundamental principles was that it considered that any organisation, grouping or stakeholder (including industry) that was likely to be affected by its decisions should be part of making those decisions. It soon became apparent that in developing its guidance development processes, one stakeholder did not appear to have a 'voice' within the NICE system. This stakeholder was the ultimate 'payer' of the NHS, the public, the taxpayer, the potential patient. Their viewpoint was likely to be very different from those of patients and their advocacy organisations seeking to gain access to every new treatment, however small the benefit.

A range of options was explored to resolve this deficit but the Citizens Council model was finally decided upon. However, this approach was not considered (nor has it been) the 'sole' means of accessing the public view, it is just one approach. During the first 10 years of its existence, NICE has used a variety of means to gain a public perspective on its work including inserting questions in national surveys, focus groups and web consultations.

It is well known that there is no one way to get the views of the public and each way has its strengths and weaknesses. What NICE wanted was a vehicle to explore what would happen when 'ordinary' people were given the time and support to delve deeply into the issues raised by having a finite health budget and ever increasing demands on that budget. Ever since the Citizens Council was established, NICE has questioned how it could be improved. The study described in Chapter 14 started the ball rolling, but every few years the NICE Board has debated whether it is the right approach, whether we should maintain it, or whether we should diversify our methods. The decision has always been that despite its shortcomings, the Citizens Council still provides a unique insight into what the public feels about the profound issues that NICE and its advisory committees face every day. Indeed it seems that many people, including

Sir Ian Kennedy in his report in July 2009,[9] consider that NICE needs to do even more to engage with the public. NICE constantly needs to describe what it does and why it is necessary. Rather than debating whether the Citizens Council should *exist*, the Board should be discussing how its role could be expanded and perhaps incorporated into a portfolio of opportunities to help the public understand the role of NICE.

The need for further evaluation and development is why the Citizens Council has remained within the Research and Development Directorate at NICE. The Citizens Council has always met in public, but the public has never really attended in any numbers. Perhaps we need to explore means of publicising the meetings and encouraging many more people to contribute to the debate.

PATIENT AND PUBLIC INVOLVEMENT – LOOKING FORWARD

Since its inception, NICE's patient and public involvement activities have adapted and expanded to accommodate NICE's rapid change and growth. As the patient and public involvement agenda gains greater importance through policy initiatives such as World Class Commissioning and service improvement and development through rapid feedback,[10] NICE continues to be at the forefront with its theoretically rigorous and pragmatic approach.

By actively and directly engaging with patients and the public at an individual and organisational level, NICE ensures that its recommendations combine a strong evidence base with the important contextual information from patient and lay experiences. This results in guidance that can be both understandable and credible to a lay audience. By improving the public's access to information about the care and treatment that should be offered to them (as outlined in NICE's guidance), NICE enables individuals to engage more actively with their healthcare professionals in shared decisions about their care. In turn, their representative organisations have more ammunition with which to lobby for the best possible care for their constituents.

NICE's multifaceted approach to patient and public involvement means it can provide useful models of engagement for those working at local, regional, national and international levels. Locally and regionally, individual health and social care organisations have obligations to appropriately involve their communities and this is driven by national policy initiatives, such as the introduction of Local Involvement Networks (LINks).[11] NICE is linking into local communities via these initiatives to encourage them to engage with NICE's guidance development implementation work.

In many ways, NICE is leading the way in patient and public involvement with links to the international guidance development community through organisations such as the Guidelines International Network (GIN)[12] and Health

Technology Assessment International (HTAi).[13] Both of these organisations have dedicated international working groups specifically promoting the patient and public involvement agenda. For many within these organisations and networks, NICE is seen as offering an exemplary service in how it engages with its lay stakeholders. Sharing NICE's considerable experience and expertise on this subject with our international colleagues, and, in turn, learning from their experiences is an excellent opportunity for all concerned to refine and further develop their strategies for patient and public involvement.

Despite the rapid pace of change during NICE's first 10 years, it has retained its reputation for rigour and transparency in its guidance development activities, and its Patient and Public Involvement Programme has always adopted the same rigorous and transparent approach to how lay people can actively engage with NICE. As we move forward into the next 10 years, we intend to build on our already strong foundations, and continue to serve as a model of good patient and public involvement.

REFERENCES

1 Department of Health. *The NHS Constitution*. London: Department of Health; 2009. Available at: www.dh.gov.uk/prod_consum_dh/groups/dh_digitalassets/documents/digitalasset/dh_093442.pdf (accessed 23 September).

2 Department of Health. *Shifting the Balance of Power: the next steps*. London: Department of Health; 2001. Available at: www.dh.gov.uk/prod_consum_dh/groups/dh_digitalassets/@dh/@en/documents/digitalasset/dh_4073554.pdf (accessed 23 September).

3 Department of Health. *Local Government and Public Involvement in Health Act 2007*. London: Office of Public Sector Information; 2006. Available at: www.opsi.gov.uk/acts/acts2007/ukpga_20070028_en_1 (accessed 23 September).

4 Department of Health. *Creating a Patient-Led NHS*. London: Department of Health; 2005. Available at: www.dh.gov.uk/assetRoot/04/10/65/07/04106507.pdf (accessed 23 September).

5 Department of Health. *Our Health, Our Care, Our Say: a new direction for community services. White paper*. London: Department of Health; 2006. Available at: www.dh.gov.uk/en/Publicationsandstatistics/Publications/PublicationsPolicyAndGuidance/DH_4127453 (accessed 23 September).

6 Bristol Inquiry Unit. *The Bristol Royal Infirmary Inquiry*. CM 5207(I). London: The Stationery Office; 2001. Available at: www.bristol-inquiry.org.uk/final_report/rpt_print.htm (accessed 23 September).

7 The BSE Inquiry. *The Inquiry into BSE and Variant CJD in the United Kingdom*. London: The Stationery Office; 2000. Available at: www.bseinquiry.gov.uk/index.htm (accessed 23 September).

8 Thomé DC. *Mid Staffordshire NHS Foundation Trust: a review of lessons learnt for commissioners and performance managers following the Healthcare Commission investigation*. London: Department of Health; 2009. Available at: www.dh.gov.uk/prod_consum_dh/groups/dh_digitalassets/documents/digitalasset/dh_098661.pdf (accessed 23 September).

9 Kennedy I. *Appraising the Value of Innovation and Other Benefits: a short study for NICE*. London: NIHCE; 2009. www.nice.org.uk/media/98F/5C/KennedyStudyFinalReport.pdf (accessed 23 September).

10 Department of Health. *Understanding What Matters: a guide to using patient feedback to transform services*. London: Department of Health; 2009. Available at: www.dh.gov.uk/prod_

consum_dh/groups/dh_digitalassets/documents/digitalasset/dh_099779.pdf (accessed 23 September).

11 Department of Health. *Listening and Responding to Communities: a brief guide to Local Involvement Networks.* London: Department of Health; 2008. Available at: www.dh.gov. uk/prod_consum_dh/groups/dh_digitalassets/@dh/@en/documents/digitalasset/ dh_087759.pdf (accessed 23 September).

12 www.g-i-n.net

13 www.htai.org

Index

Abélard, Pierre 165
access to treatments
    innovation value appraisals 107–8
    intervention thresholds 106–7
    'only-in-research' recommendations 102–4
accountability and reasonableness 139–46
advisory committee meetings *see* public
    advisory body meetings
age and levels of care 119–20
    Citizens Council (NICE) reports 91–2
age-related macular degeneration (AMD) 37
anecdotal evidence from patients *see* patient
    evidence
appeals 142
attitudes of patients and the public *see* social
    value judgements
awareness-raising campaigns 61

Baker, Professor Richard 12
behaviour-dependent conditions 120
bioethical principles 110–12
biological therapies, targeted 37
buddy schemes 68

Care Quality Commission 6–7
CEA *see* cost-effectiveness analysis (CEA)
    methodologies
charities 42–3
choice *see* patient choice
Citizens Council (NICE) 5, 71, 75–80
    aims of PPIP 83
    dealing with challenges and critiques
      133–5
    demographic characteristics 79
    evaluating effectiveness 145–6
    functions 11
    future concerns and considerations 183–4
    importance of public perspectives 127–8
    membership and remuneration 77–8
    opportunities for involvement 11
      comments and findings 11–12
    outcomes and reflections 79–80

personal accounts and experiences 125–8
on public health guidance 40
question setting 84
recruitment and engagement 78–9, 81–3,
    130–1
reports 89–108
role of facilitators 132
setting up dilemmas and experiences
    129–38
tips and advice 130–8
topic choice and agendas 85–6
see also Citizens Council (NICE) Reports
Citizens Council (NICE) Reports 89–108
    1st – Clinical Need 90–1
    2nd – Age 91–2
    3rd – Confidential Enquiries 92–5
    4th – Ultra-Orphan Drugs 95–6
    5th – Mandatory Public Health Measures
      96–100
    6th – Rule of Rescue 100–1
    7th – Health Inequalities 101–2
    8th – Research 102–4
    9th – Patient Safety 104–5
    10th – QALY and illness severity 105–6
    11th – Intervention Thresholds 106–7
    12th – Value of Innovations 107–8
clinical guidelines (NICE) 2, 19–26
    bodies and groups involved 19
    consultation and production methods 20
    development of 'short time-scale'
      programmes 16, 20
    involvement of patients and carers 20–6
      aims and rationale 20–1
      methods of engagement 21–2
      support measures 21
    publication and implementation issues 26
    responses to draft proposals 25
    role of commercial organisations 22
    role of patient evidence 24
    scope and remits 22
    terminology and language use 25
    use of development groups (GDGs) 23–4